SNAKE OIL
And Other Preoccupations

John Diamond died on March 2nd 2001. He was one of Britain's most prolific journalists, columnists and broadcasters, having worked for most of the national papers and presented numerous radio and television series. He was married to Nigella Lawson, with whom he had two children.

Dominic Lawson is Editor of the *Sunday Telegraph*. Previously he was Editor of the *Spectator*. He introduced John Diamond as a columnist at both titles. He was also John Diamond's brother-in-law.

ALSO BY JOHN DIAMOND
C: Because Cowards Get Cancer Too

John Diamond

SNAKE OIL
And Other Preoccupations

INTRODUCTION BY
Dominic Lawson

FOREWORD BY
Richard Dawkins

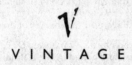

VINTAGE

Published by Vintage 2001

2 4 6 8 10 9 7 5 3 1

Copyright © John Diamond 2001
Introduction © Dominic Lawson 2001
Foreword © Richard Dawkins 2001

Grateful acknowledgment is made to the *Daily Mail*, *Jewish Chronicle*, *Observer*, *She*, *Spectator*, *Sunday Telegraph*, *Sunday Telegraph Magazine*, *Sunday Times*, *Sunday Times Magazine* and *The Times Magazine* for permission to reproduce the articles within this collection.

First published in Great Britain in 2001 by Vintage

Vintage
Random House, 20 Vauxhall Bridge Road, London SW1V 2SA
Random House Australia (Pty) Limited
20 Alfred Street, Milsons Point, Sydney,
New South Wales 2061, Australia

Random House New Zealand Limited
18 Poland Road, Glenfield, Auckland 10, New Zealand

Random House South Africa (Pty) Limited
Endulini, 5A Jubilee Road, Parktown 2193, South Africa

Random House UK Limited Reg. No. 954009
www.randomhouse.co.uk

A CIP catalogue record for this book
is available from the British Library

ISBN 0 09 942833 4

A VINTAGE ORIGINAL

Papers used by Random House UK Ltd are natural, recyclable products made from wood grown in sustainable forests. The manufacturing processes conform to the environmental regulations of the country of origin

Set in 10½/12 Sabon by SX Composing DTP, Rayleigh, Essex
Printed and bound in Great Britain by
Bookmarque Ltd, Croydon, Surrey

Contents

INTRODUCTION

DOMINIC LAWSON

When one thinks of the pain John Diamond must have felt at leaving the world when his two children were so young, it seems almost tasteless to suggest that his departure before completing 'an uncomplimentary view of complementary medicine' – as he dubbed his book – was also a tragedy. But the editor in me, as opposed to the brother-in-law, certainly does see it as that. John's study on the day after his death presented an almost unbearably poignant sight: his computer screen still switched on, and there, flickering, as if with an extinguished intelligence, the last completed words of his book before he was rushed to hospital: 'Let me explain.' For once, he never did.

In that study, too, could be found almost every word that John had ever written, torn out of the myriad newspapers and magazines to which he had contributed, before cyberspace developed an easier means of retrieval. Six months before he died John wrote that he had rejected requests to set up a website devoted to his articles because 'I've always believed that journalism is an ephemeral thing and that if I want to write anything for posterity's sake, I'll start another unfinishable book.' But the sight of that pile of accumulated cuttings in the study suggested to Nigella and me that perhaps John would actually have relished seeing the best of it between covers: smarter than a mere website, in any event.

We are both grateful to Zöe Wales and Sally Duncan for their help in collating all of John's journalism: he was the archetypal freelance, prepared to write about anything for anyone, so theirs was not an easy task. Actually, this was never mere hackery on his part. John had absorbed more information, both useful and useless, about a wider range of subjects, than any other journalist I came across. The Internet, fashion, cars, restaurants, television: on all these topics he at one time or another (and frequently simultaneously) had regular columns. John had an almost unerring sense of what the latest 'thing' would be in all these fields, and had a fierce desire to share his discoveries with as many people as possible. He was, for example, the first television critic to spot the peculiar talent of Sacha Baron-Cohen, languishing on the Paramount Comedy Channel, so that the readers of the *Sunday Telegraph* became the perhaps unlikely avant-garde fan club of the man who subsequently gained greater fame as Ali G.

I joined John Diamond's fan club in January 1989 when, showing a courage bordering on the reckless, he agreed to write a travel piece for the *Spectator* on Geneva, one of the most boring of the world's great cities. He turned this unfortunate fact into a piece of irresistible wit: 'Whole streets in the centre of town go bank, Rolex, bank, bank, Patek Philippe, bank, bank, Japanese electronics store, bank, bank, bank, Longines, greengrocer, Omega, bank, bank, bank.'

I remember ringing Nigella up, knowing that she was then a colleague of John's at the *Sunday Times*, to read out loud and share with her the only funny piece (so far as I know) ever to have been written about Geneva. I couldn't have been happier when, three months or so later, Nigella's office friendship with John turned into something much more precious.

John's gift of humour was certainly what I treasured most as one of his many editors – he was writing five columns a week at the time of his death. He was, as his obituarists wrote, an incredibly witty man in private conversation (even when deprived of speech, and forced to scribble his repartee). But we all know writers who are outrageously witty in private, yet who struggle to realise that comic timing in their writing. Conversely, there are many very funny writers who in their real lives are models only of misanthropy. With John the wit was seamless, without force or contrivance. This remained true, right to the very end, even when he was in constant physical pain: you don't have to be Jewish, although, as they say, it helps, to be reduced to helpless laughter by his *Jewish Chronicle* swansong, a mock-Yiddisher version of 'Twas the week before Christmas'.

John's Jewishness was not just the wellspring of much of his sense of humour (if the Jews are a race, then irony is definitely its common language); it was also the object of his wit. His column in *The Times* contained some wonderful examples, none better than his account (included here) of a profoundly embarrassing trip to a Hasidim-run computer repair shop.

John's column in *The Times* became, I suppose, his public memorial, with its frequently (and deliberately) poignant account of the havoc wrought by a smoking-induced tumour. It was the intensely personal tone of these columns which clearly captured the attention of so many readers. But their strength, it seems to me (and to many doctors as well, to judge from the letters sent in at the time of John's death), rests in large part with his absolute determination to understand the true nature of his disease, and to communicate that, rather than mere emotion, to his readers. John's family background – his father had been a bio-chemist – obviously helped, but this was also characteristic of him as a writer: unlike so many prolific and gifted columnists he never allowed himself to run on a tank full only of treasured prejudices. He certainly had those, too, but above all he was an empirical writer, obsessed, as all seekers of truth are, with facts, facts, facts. Readers rather enjoy that, by the way: on the whole, that's why people buy newspapers.

One of John's readers wrote to *The Times* in the week of his death, arguing that while his columns on his illness were being much praised, his gifts as a humorous writer were in danger of being forgotten. I think that was a shrewd judgement, and it explains why I have tried to make this selection on the basis of his humour rather than his tumour.

As for the latter (damn it to hell) it is important not to fall for the idea that John's 'Diary of Courage' – as it was sometimes headlined, much to his irritation – was a complete opening of his soul to his readers. His skill lay in convincing his readers that this was a true confessional across which they had stumbled: in fact, his public never knew just how black his moods could become, how great his physical pain, how deep his mental torment. The John Diamond in those columns was in part an idealised version of himself, designed to help him cope with his illness, but which also must have hugely lifted the spirits of readers who were in the grip of this foul disease, or who had relatives in that predicament.

This is not, by the way, a criticism of John, either as a columnist or as a person: writing is an art, more than a science, and to have been in reality as insouciant as the columnar Diamond was about his predicament – well, that would have been less than fully human. And as humans go, they don't come much fuller than John Diamond.

Dallington, April 2001

FOREWORD

RICHARD DAWKINS

John Diamond gave short shrift to those among his many admirers who praised his courage. But there are distinct kinds of courage, and we mustn't confuse them. There's physical fortitude in the face of truly outrageous fortune, the stoical courage to endure pain and indignity while wrestling heroically with a peculiarly nasty form of cancer. Diamond disclaimed this kind of courage for himself (I think too modestly, and in any case nobody could deny the equivalent in his wonderful wife). He even used the subtitle *Because Cowards Get Cancer Too* for his moving and I still think brave memoir of his own affliction.

But there's another kind of courage, and here John Diamond is unequivocally up there with the best of them. This is intellectual courage: the courage to stick by your intellectual principles, even when *in extremis* and sorely tempted by the easy solace that a betrayal might seem to offer. From Socrates through David Hume to today, those led by reason to eschew the security blanket of irrational superstition have always been challenged: 'It's fine for you to talk like that now. Just wait till you are on your deathbed. You'll soon change your tune.' The solace politely refused by Hume (as we know from Boswell's morbidly curious deathbed visit) was one appropriate to his time. In John Diamond's time, and ours, it is 'alternative' miracle cures, offered when orthodox medicine seems to be failing and may even have given up on us.

When the pathologist has read the runes; when the oracles of X-ray, CT scan and biopsy have spoken and hope is guttering low; when the surgeon enters the room accompanied by 'a tallish man . . . looking embarrassed . . . in hood and gown with a scythe over his shoulder', it is then that the 'alternative' or 'complementary' vultures start circling. This is their moment. This is where they come into their own, for there's money in hope: the more desperate the hope, the richer the pickings. And, to be fair, many pushers of dishonest remedies are motivated by an honest desire to help. Their persistent importunings of the gravely ill, their intrusively urgent offers of pills and potions, have a sincerity that rises above the financial greed of the quacks they promote.

Have you tried squid's cartilage? Establishment doctors scorn it, of course, but my aunt is still alive on squid's cartilage two years after her oncologist gave her only six months (well, yes, since you ask, she is having radio-therapy as *well*). Or there's this wonderful healer who practises the laying on of feet, with astonishing results. Apparently it's all a question of tuning your holistic (or is it holographic?) energies to the natural frequencies of organic (or is it orgonic?) cosmic vibrations. You've nothing to lose, you might as well try it. It's £500 for a course of treatment, which may sound a lot but what's money when your life is at stake?

As a public figure who wrote, movingly and personally, about the horrible progress of his cancer, John Diamond was more than usually exposed to such siren songs: actively inundated with well-intentioned advice and offers of miracles. He examined the claims, looked for evidence in their favour, found none, saw further that the false hopes they aroused could actually be damaging – and he retained this honesty and clarity of vision to the end. When my time comes, I do not expect to show a quarter of John Diamond's physical forti-tude, disavow it though he might. But I very much hope to use him as my model when it comes to intellectual courage.

The obvious and immediate counter charge is one of arrogance. Far from being rational, wasn't John Diamond's 'intellectual courage' really an unreasoning overconfidence in science, a blind and bigoted refusal to contemplate alternative views of the world, and of human health? No, no and no. The accusation would stick if he had bet on orthodox medicine simply because it is orthodox, and shunned alternative medicine simply because it is alternative. But of course he did no such thing. For his purposes (and mine), scientific medicine is *defined* as the set of practices which submit themselves to the ordeal of being *tested*. Alternative medicine is defined as that set of practices which cannot be tested, refuse to be tested, or consistently fail tests. If a healing technique is demonstrated to have curative properties in properly controlled double-blind trials, it ceases to be alternative. It simply, as Diamond explains, becomes medicine. Conversely, if a technique devised by the President of the Royal College of Physicians consistently fails in double-blind trials, it will cease to be a part of 'orthodox' medicine. Whether it will then become 'alternative' will depend upon whether it is adopted by a sufficiently ambitious quack (there are always sufficiently gullible patients).

But isn't it still an arrogance to demand that our method of testing should be the scientific method? By all means use scientific tests for scientific medicine, it may be said. But isn't it only fair that 'alternative' medicine should be tested by 'alternative' tests? No. There is no such thing as an alternative test. Here Diamond takes his stand, and he is right to do so. Either it is true that a medicine works or it isn't. It cannot be false in the ordinary sense but true in some 'alternative' sense. If a therapy or treatment is anything more than a placebo, properly conducted double-blind trials, statistically analysed, will eventually bring it through with flying colours. Many candidates for recognition as 'orthodox' medicines fail the test and are summarily dropped. The 'alternative' label should not (though, alas, it does) provide immunity from the same fate.

Prince Charles has recently called for ten million pounds of government money to be spent researching the claims of 'alternative' or 'complementary' medicine. An admirable suggestion, although it is not immediately clear why government, which has to juggle competing priorities, is the appropriate source of money, given that the leading 'alternative' techniques have already been tested – and have failed – again and again and again. John Diamond tells us that the alternative medicine business in Britain has a turnover measured in billions of pounds. Perhaps some small fraction of the profits generated by these medicines could be diverted into testing whether they actually work. This, after all, is what 'orthodox' pharmaceutical companies are expected to do. Could it be that purveyors of alternative medicine know all too well what the upshot of properly conducted trials would be? If so, their reluctance to fund their own nemesis is all too understandable. Nevertheless, I hope this research money will come from somewhere, perhaps from Prince Charles's own charitable resources, and I would be happy to serve on an advisory committee to disburse it, if invited to do so. Actually, I suspect that ten million pounds' worth of research is more than would be necessary to see off most of the more popular and lucrative 'alternative' practices.

How might the money be spent? Let's take homeopathy as an example, and let us suppose that we have a large enough fraction of the grant to plan the experiment on a moderately large scale. Having given their consent, 1,000 patients will be separated into 500 experimentals (who will receive the homeopathic dose) and 500 controls (who will not). Bending over backwards to respect the 'holistic' principle that every individual must be treated as an individual, we shall not insist on giving all experimental subjects the same dose. Nothing so crude. Instead, every patient in the trial shall be examined by a certified homeopath, and an individually tailored therapy prescribed. The different patients need not even receive the same homeopathic substance.

But now comes the all-important double-blind randomisation. After every patient's prescription has been written, half of the patients, at random, will be designated controls. The controls will not in fact receive their prescribed dose. Instead, they will be given a dose which is identified only by impenetrable code numbers. This is vitally important because nobody denies the placebo effect: patients who think they are getting an effective cure feel better than patients who think the opposite.

Each patient will be examined by a team of doctors and homeopaths, both before and after the treatment. This team will write down their judgement for each patient: has this patient got better, stayed the same, or got worse? Only when these verdicts have all been written down and sealed will the randomising codes in the computer be broken. Only then will we know which patients had received the homeopathic dose and which the control placebo. The results will be analysed statistically to see whether the homeopathic doses had any effect, one way or the other. I know which result my shirt is on, but – this is the beauty of good science – I cannot bias the outcome. Nor can the homeopaths who are betting on the opposite. The double-blind experimental design disempowers all such biases. The experiment can be performed by advocates or sceptics, or both working together, and it won't change the result.

There are all sorts of details by which this experimental design could be made more sensitive. The patients could be sorted into 'matched pairs', matched for age, weight, sex, diagnosis, prognosis and preferred homeopathic prescription. The only consistent difference is that one member of each pair is randomly and secretly designed a control, and given a placebo. The statistics then specifically compare each experimental individual with his matched control.

The ultimate matched-pairs design is to use each patient as his own control, receiving the experimental and the control dose successively, and never knowing when the change occurs. The order of administering the two treatments to a given patient would be determined at random, a different random schedule for different patients.

'Matched pairs' and 'own control' experimental designs have the advantage of increasing the sensitivity of the test. Increasing, in other words, the chance of yielding a statistically significant success for homeopathy. Notice that a statistically significant success is not a very demanding criterion. It is not necessary that every patient should feel better on the homeopathic dose than on the control. All we are looking for is a slight advantage to homeopathy over the blind control, an advantage which, however slight, is too great to be attributable to luck, according to the standard methods of statistics. This is what is routinely demanded of orthodox medicines before they are allowed to be advertised and sold as curative. It is rather less than is demanded by a prudent pharmaceutical company before it will invest a lot of money in mass production.

Now we come to an awkward fact about homeopathy in particular, dealt with in the book itself, but worth stressing here. It is a fundamental tenet of homeopathic theory that the active ingredient – arnica, bee venom, or whatever it is – must be successively diluted some large number of times, until – all calculations agree – there is not a single molecule of that ingredient remaining. Indeed, homeopaths make the daringly paradoxical claim that the *more* dilute the solution the *more* potent its action. The investigative conjuror James Randi has calculated that, after a typical sequence of homeopathic 'successive' dilutions, there would be one molecule of active ingredient in a vat the size of the solar system! (Actually, in practice, there will be more stray molecules than the desired homeopathic dose knocking around even in water of the highest attainable purity.)

Now, think what this does. The whole rationale of the experiment is to compare experimental doses (which include the active ingredient) with control doses (which include all the same ingredients except the active one). The two doses must look the same, taste the same, feel the same in the mouth. The only respect in which they differ must be the presence or absence of the putatively curative ingredient. But in the case of homeopathic medicine, the dilution is such that there is no difference between the experimental dose and the control! Both contain the same number of molecules of the active ingredient – zero, or whatever is the minimum attainable in practice. This seems to suggest that a double-blind trial of homeopathy cannot, in principle, succeed. You could even say that a successful result would be diagnostic of a failure to dilute sufficiently!

There is a conceivable loophole, much slithered through by homeopaths ever since this embarrassing difficulty was brought to their attention. The mode of action of their remedies, they say, is not chemical but physical. They agree that not a single molecule of the active ingredient remains in the bottle that you buy, but this only matters if you insist on thinking chemically. They believe that, by some physical mechanism unknown to physicists, a kind of 'trace' or 'memory' of the active molecules is imprinted on the water molecules used to dilute them. It is the physically imprinted template on the water that cures the patient, not the chemical nature of the original ingredient.

This is a respectable scientific hypothesis in the sense that it is testable. Easy to test, indeed, and although I wouldn't bother to test it myself, this is only because I think our finite supply of time and money would be better spent testing something more plausible. But any homeopath who really believes his theory should be beavering away from dawn to dusk. After all, if the double-blind trials of patient treatments came out reliably and repeatably positive, he would win a Nobel Prize not only in Medicine but in Physics as well. He would have discovered a brand-new principle of physics, perhaps a new fundamental force in the universe. With such a prospect in view, homeopaths must surely be falling over each other in their eagerness to be first into the lab, racing like alternative Watsons and Cricks to claim this glittering scientific crown. Er, actually no they aren't. Can it be that they don't really believe their theory after all?

At this point we scrape the barrel of excuses. 'Some things are true on a human level, but they don't lend themselves to scientific testing. The sceptical atmosphere of the science lab is not conducive to the sensitive forces involved.' Such excuses are commonly trotted out by practitioners of alternative therapies, including those that don't have homeopathy's peculiar difficulties of principle but which nevertheless consistently fail to pass double-blind tests in practice. John Diamond is a pungently witty writer, and one of the funniest passages of this book is his description of an experimental test of 'kinesiology' by Ray Hyman, my colleague on CSICOP (the Committee for the Scientific Investigation of Claims of the Paranormal).

As it happens, I have personal experience of kinesiology. It was used by the one quack practitioner I have – to my shame – consulted. I had ricked my neck. A therapist specialising in manipulation had been strongly recommended. Manipulation can undoubtedly be very effective, and this woman was available at the weekend, when I didn't like to trouble my normal doctor. Pain and an open mind drove me to give her a try. Before she began the manipulation itself, her diagnostic technique was kinesiology. I had to lie down and stretch out my arm, and she pushed against it, testing my strength. The key to the diagnosis was the effect of vitamin C on my arm-wrestling performance. But I wasn't asked to imbibe the vitamin. Instead (I am not exaggerating, this is the literal truth), a sealed bottle containing vitamin C was placed on my chest. This appeared to cause an immediate and dramatic increase in the strength of my arm, pushing against hers. When I expressed my natural scepticism, she said happily, 'Yes, C is a *marvellous* vitamin, isn't it!' Human politeness stopped me walking out there and then, and I even (to avoid hassle) ended up paying her lousy fee.

What was needed (I doubt if that woman would even have understood the point) was a series of double blind trials, in which neither she nor I was allowed to know whether the bottle contained the alleged active ingredient or something else. This was what Professor Hyman, in John Diamond's hilarious description of a similar case, undertook. I won't spoil the story by repeating it here, but let me just call attention to the ludicrous response of the kinesiologist when, as one would expect, his method ignominiously flunked the double blind test (page 68).

A large part of the history of science, especially medical science, has been a progressive weaning away from the superficial seductiveness of individual stories which seem – but only seem – to show a pattern. The human mind is a wanton storyteller and, even more, a profligate seeker after pattern. We see faces in clouds and tortillas, fortunes in tea leaves and planetary movements. It is quite difficult to prove a real pattern, as distinct from a superficial illusion. The human mind has to learn to mistrust its native tendency to run away with itself and see pattern where there is only randomness. That is what statistics are for, and that is why no drug of therapeutic technique should be adopted until it has been proved by a statistically analysed experiment, in which the fallible pattern-seeking proclivities of the human mind have been systematically taken out of the picture. Personal stories are never good evidence for any general trend.

In spite of this, doctors have been heard to begin a judgement with something like, 'The trials all say otherwise, but in *my* clinical experience . . .' This might constitute better grounds for changing your doctor than a suable malpractice! That, at least, would seem to follow from all that I have been saying. But it is an exaggeration. Certainly, before a medicine is certified for wide use, it must be properly tested and given the imprimatur of statistical significance. But a mature doctor's clinical experience is at least an excellent guide to which hypotheses might be worth going to the trouble and expense of testing. And there's more that can be said. Rightly or wrongly (often rightly) we actually do take the personal judgement of a respected human individual seriously. This is obviously so with aesthetic judgements, which is why a famous critic can make or break a play on Broadway or Shaftesbury Avenue. Whether we like it or not, people are swayed by anecdote, by the particular, by the personal.

And this, almost paradoxically, helps to make John Diamond such a powerful advocate. He is a man whom we like and admire for his personal story, and whose opinions we want to read because he expresses them so well. People who might not listen to a set of nameless statistics, intoned by a faceless scientist or doctor, will listen to John Diamond, not just because he writes engagingly, but because he was dying while he wrote and he knew it: dying in spite of the best efforts of the very medical practices he was defending against opponents whose only weapon is anecdote. But there is really no paradox. He may gain our ear because of his singular qualities and his human story. But what we hear when we listen to him is not anecdotal. It stands up to rigorous examination. It would be sensible and compelling in its own right even if its author had not previously earned our admiration and our affection.

John Diamond was never going to go gentle into that good night. When he did go it was with guns blazing, for the splendidly polemical chapters now before you occupied him right up to the end, working against . . . not so much the clock as time's wingèd chariot itself. He does not rage against the dying of the light, nor against his wicked cancer, nor against cruel fate. What would be the point, for what would they care? His targets are capable of wincing when hit. They are targets that deserve to be hit hard, targets whose neutralisation would leave the world a better place: cynical charlatans (or honestly foolish dreamers) who prey on gullible unfortunates. And the best part is that although this gallant man is dead, his guns are not silenced. He left a strong emplacement. This posthumous book launches his broadside, and it is about to be published. Open fire, and don't stop.

Oxford, April 2001

SNAKE OIL

CHAPTER ONE

WHAT FOLLOWS IS not a defence of orthodox medicine any more than a book attacking, say, Marxism would necessarily be a defence of global capitalism. I've not written it because I think the multinational pharmaceutical companies are ethical paragons, or because I believe the medical establishment isn't capable of being self-serving, hidebound and inflexible. I know that there are any number of things which your pharmacist can give you which will kill you and that there are some hospitals in Britain where you are almost guaranteed to leave in a worse state than you were when you were admitted. I could write about that medical establishment or those lousy hospitals, but there are plenty of books around on the practical and philosophical failings of the medical orthodoxy and precious few on the failings of alternative medicine.

Which is surprising given that alternative medicine in Britain is a business with a turnover of billions of pounds and an establishment all of its own, a business which gets regular and often uncritical coverage in most of our popular papers and magazines, which regularly makes – or allows to be made on its behalf – remarkable claims for its abilities, which are often untested, let alone proven, which has no independent body monitoring its activities and which from time to time kills its customers as a direct result of the advice or actions of its practitioners.

Science, which was going to save us all in the Sixties, gets a pretty bad press these days. It's not just because science has been the tool used to discover the principles behind the atomic bomb or the atmosphere-clogging internal combustion engine, although there is that too. But all too often the pundits treat science as if it were just one of a number of equivalent techniques for gaining new knowledge. The suggestion is rather that just as an architect may choose between brick and stone for his building, and make that choice using various established criteria which tell him that brick works best here and concrete there, so somebody in the healing game charged with testing the validity of a remedy may choose to use science to do the job or then again use . . . well, what? Instinct? Faith? A hunch? Dice?

All of which is to ignore what science is. It isn't one particular way of ascertaining a physical truth: by definition it is *the* way of ascertaining physical truth. Or, more accurately, try it the other way around: anything which discovers or proves such a truth is science. But then truth is a pretty vague term these days too. Many of the alternative practitioners I've talked to over the years get to the bit of the argument (and invariably it's an argument if I'm there) where the truth of their premise comes into question and they smile and say, 'Ah! Truth! Well, it depends what you mean . . .'*

But the truth is that most of us know just what we mean by truth. We test out the laws of physics and chemistry a thousand, a million times a day without thinking about them, and find them to be true. Every breath we take, every beat of our heart, every blink of our eye is a demonstration of any

---

* And a warm welcome to visiting post-modernists. Yes, I know there are a number of interesting theories about the invalidity of scientific proof, based on the premise that because facts exist only as a function of fallible human perception, modified by our fallible human senses, they can never be 'known' in the way a scientist would claim to know them. And I know those same post-modernist theorists would claim that the facts of science as understood by Pacific-Island animists or members of the Flat Earth Society are just as valid as the facts of science as understood by the President of the Royal Society. Go ahead. Theorise. You'll find no argument against those theses in this book, nor any acknowledgement of them beyond this footnote. This is a book about truth as the vast majority of the population – including most alternativists – would understand it rather than a discussion of competing philosophies. Sorry.

number of physical truths. And we accept those truths whenever we step on to the floor without worrying about whether *this* time the atoms of our foot will become confused with the atoms of the floorboards and we'll slip through to the room below. Newton's laws are demonstrated every time our arm muscles tighten minutely in response to the weight of the door we're opening, Ohm's laws every time we switch on the light without worrying that the electricity will slip through the plastic of the switch and electrocute us.

And that is what science is – all it is, indeed. It's trying things out to see what happens, and discovering that those things which happen over and over again are true. If I hit a nail with a hammer in precisely the same way a hundred, a thousand, a million times, then not even the most laid-back anti-scientist could very well argue that this doesn't tell us something about the indisputable physical nature of steel and wood and the expenditure and conversion of energy. And in the same way, if I take a million people with a headache and give them an aspirin and the headache goes away, this demonstrates a truth about the chemical interaction of aspirin with the brain's pain receptors.

Of course, as both orthodox and alternative practitioners will point out, we get headaches for any number of different reasons and one man's throbbing hangover is another's growing brain tumour. If the science of determining the truth about the ways of the human body – not to say the ways of the human mind – were as easy as determining the physics involved in hammering in a nail to put up a picture, then there wouldn't be much left for medical researchers to do. But the body is complicated, the brain more complicated still and, as any holistic believer will tell you, few illnesses are about easily diagnosed malfunctions of single bits of the body. If medical science were like hammer-and-nail science then the cure rates for various illnesses would all be either 100 per cent or zero: yes, we know how to cure tuberculosis and so all tuberculosis is cured; no, we haven't yet worked out how to cure cancer so all cancer patients die. The reality is that we've worked out what causes tuberculosis and what will kill the TB bacillus, but still people catch the disease and still some people die of it, and still new forms of it appear and demand we find new forms of the old treatments; we have rather less idea of what causes many cancers, but still we have medical techniques which cure some patients, give others a longer lease of life and consign others still to a cancerous death.

Which is probably the point where I should point out precisely which axes I shall be grinding over the following pages.

I'm not a doctor, and I'm not even a scientist, although I come from a vaguely scientific family where the disciplines of scientific endeavour were made clear to me at a fairly early age. Then again, most alternative practitioners aren't doctors and many are proud in their rejection of what most scientists would regard as conventional science. I'm a journalist. Four years ago, as I write, I contracted cancer of the throat and used the column I write in *The Times* to describe the medical and practical effects of the cancer and its treatment. As the story of my treatment – surgery, radiotherapy, chemotherapy, all undertaken at a London cancer hospital under the guidance of various medical luminaries – unrolled on the page week after week, so mail started arriving from readers who thought I was committing long-term suicide by consigning my cancer to orthodox medicine and that I would be better off taking one of a number of alternative routes. I should, they said, take Essiac, the treatment of preference for members of Native American tribes in Canada, or I should try homeopathy or Laetrile or vitamin C and zinc. They sent me the addresses of clinics just across the Mexican border from California where renegade doctors would charge me $20,000 a week to treat my cancer with substances and methods banned in the US, and they sent newsletters from organisations promoting the use of coffee-ground enemas to cure cancer.

Most of these messages were sent with the best and most generous of intentions and I wish I could tell you that I read them with a mind entirely open to the promises they offered. But this wasn't the first time I'd come across alternative remedies.

Fifteen years earlier I went through one of the routine bouts of vague and minor mental and physical distress which strike most men as they slip out of young manhood and into that age where life's possibilities seem suddenly more limited. I started turning up regularly at my GP's surgery with a list of those ailments which, it turns out, make up most of the average city-centre GP's case-load: inexplicable tiredness, lethargy, various non-specific aches and pains, unwonted anxieties. Like most patients presenting these sorts of symptom, I was certain they were the result of some specific organic illness and was annoyed when the doctor looked at the blood tests and the ECG results and the hospital reports and couldn't find evidence of the specific illness I knew must be lurking there. What I needed was somebody to tell me to stop working fifteen-hour days and playing twelve-hour nights; what I wanted the doctor to say was, 'Ah! Chronic Farnsbarns Syndrome! Take this linctus twice a day for a week and you'll feel better again.'

With the orthodoxy failing to come up with a solution, I did what so many of us do these days: I looked for an alternative answer. I started buying paperback books with titles like *The Stone Age Diet* and *Understanding Your Allergies*. Invariably the books would have an introductory chapter, which would list the symptoms which result from not eating the diet that our Stone Age forebears had eaten, or from being allergic to any number of normal foods – including, of course, those which our Stone Age forebears had eaten. And what do you know? Every one of my symptoms was there: lassitude, aching bones, anxiety, odd bouts of melancholy . . . I had found the answer. Of course the lists didn't just include my own symptoms: they included every non-specific symptom you could imagine. Anyone reading the books would find their imagined illnesses described (and I'll grant that an illness is no less distressing or intractable just because it's imagined) as, more worryingly, would those with organic illnesses needing real treatment.

As a rationalist I tried to make these book-based diagnoses seem equally rational. I had to strain at my own credulity, but I managed. Of *course* my diet was wrong: my prehistoric forebears had lived off nuts and grains rather than meat pies and chips and it stood to reason that my system would be overloaded by the modern diet. Never mind that one of the wonders of human physiology is the sheer range of fuels on which we can run happily: just ask the Inuit who has never seen a field of wheat and lives on a diet of fish and whale blubber, or the Australian bushman hundreds of miles from the nearest coastline living on nuts, berries and meat. And of *course* I was allergic: hay fever had sabotaged my summer for the first time when I was thirty, so why could it not be that I'd suddenly developed allergies to something other than pollen?

I changed my diet to one of rice crackers and peanut butter, and for a week or two lived a new and self-regarding life which seemed slightly freer of the symptoms. Until they returned. So I phoned a number in the allergy book and was directed to a man in Bayswater who called himself a clinical ecologist and claimed to be able to detect all sorts of allergies using new and scientific means. Not only did he have a scientific basis for his allergy theories, but he was a real scientist – a man with a doctorate in pharmacology from a proper British university – whose theories about allergies, their detection and cure, seemed at first glance reasonable. After various tests he gave me a list of the things I was allergic to: tangerines but not oranges, Brussels sprouts but no other member of the brassica family, a few other common foods which I ate regularly and which were, he said, upsetting my system.

In one sense this isn't alternative medicine: orthodox medicine also recognises allergies, tests for them (but not using the methods of my clinical ecologist) and usually gives much the same cure as he did, which is to avoid eating the stuff to which I was supposedly allergic.

My clinical ecologist was part of a substratum of alternative medicine, for while one part of the industry tries to dissociate itself from 'real' science and happily accepts the stereotypical image which has a bean-bag replacing an examination table, there is another section which likes to think of itself as scientific in the real sense of the word, using accepted scientific rules to try to justify theories which the medical mainstream hasn't yet got round to accepting.

Indeed, my practitioner went one stage further than offering an alternative diagnostic method or an alternative treatment: he found a whole alternative illness.

There are a few of these around and very often they are real illnesses. What makes them 'alternative' is that while orthodox medicine detects them in a few or very few cases, alternative medicine finds them all over the place. The most well known, I suppose, is ME or myalgic encephalomyelitis, or as it was known when it first hit the headlines in the Seventies, Yuppie Flu. The symptoms of ME are precisely those vaguely defined ones which appear in the alternative books on diet and allergy, and while some orthodox doctors recognise the illness, and some believe it to be, at best, a collective name for a number of other illnesses with similar symptoms, it's a diagnosis you'll rarely hear given in an orthodox surgery. But there are alternative therapists who claim to diagnose it in almost any patient who presents with those vague, headachey tired symptoms I had, and its great advantage as far as alternative medicine is concerned is that, while the orthodoxy might grudgingly acknowledge it, they also acknowledge that the only possible diagnosis is a clinical one. That is to say that there is no blood or any other test which will conclusively show the presence of the ME virus (although some, who refer to it as post-viral fatigue syndrome would argue with that – but I'm getting way ahead of myself here) and diagnosis depends on the patient's symptoms. True, there are examples of people who have incapacitating symptoms which take them to bed for years at a time and which some orthodox doctors accept is the result of ME, but these are rarities.

In many ways it's the perfect modern alternative illness. It has an impressive name, explains the presence of all those symptoms which stop you enjoying work and home life as much as you think you ought to, or as much as you believe everyone else does, and gives its sufferers a good medical reason to do that which they probably ought to do anyway: get to bed earlier, lay off the booze, eat a little more carefully, work less fervently.

There are other such illnesses which alternativists claim to be able to find where the orthodoxy can't, including a few that supposedly result from various nutritional deficiencies, which go some way to explain the piles of vitamin and mineral supplements on the shelves of your local branch of Boots.

9

In fact, according to my man I had none of these: what I had was another alternative favourite – an infestation of the yeast-like fungus *candida* in my gut. Again, no test of the contents of my stomach was ever made, no sample ever taken: this was a clinical diagnosis. The treatment was midway between alternative and orthodox, which is to say that there was a sort of brazen logic to the treatment which involved drinking a powdered version of the stuff that women with a yeast infection of their vagina use on themselves. Wouldn't you know it: the stuff had to be imported from California and cost a fortune.

Again, for a couple of weeks I felt better, and then to celebrate how much better I was feeling I started working the long days and stumbling through the long nights again, and sure enough, the symptoms returned. It wasn't until I learned to calm down, rest properly, drink less, eat more sensibly, work with more regard to my own well-being and less regard to promotion, that the symptoms started to disappear for good.

At the time I spent much of my professional life as a consumer journalist on the *Sunday Times Magazine* and found myself writing more and more often about consumer medicine and in particular, and as a result of my experience in Bayswater, alternative medicine. It was the start of the boom in alternativism – not only as the province of the practitioners of the established therapies, but by the big commercial companies, which used the principles and philosophies of alternativism to sell their products. It was the age when alternative remedies started appearing on the shelves of the high-street pharmacy chain stores, an age of the coming of, for instance, Aqua Libra – remember that? – a soft drink which promoted itself by claiming to correct the alkalinity of the overstressed modern body – a view of the body and its workings which ignored the facts of basic human physiology in a way that would have made any iridologist or reflexologist proud.

But then it was also the height of Thatcherism, and while I don't want to get too precious about the essential philosophy behind alternativism, and while I realise the average alternative and liberal-minded therapist would be horrified by the comparison, it's no coincidence that alternative medicine grew as Margaret Thatcher's *Weltanschauung* took hold. In many ways it was where the fading hippiedom of the early Seventies was able to meet the new materialism of the Thatcherites head-on. Alternative medicine, like Thatcherism, tells us that our personal well-being is entirely in our own hands, that we can all have anything we want – perfect health, freedom from anxiety – if we want it *enough* and are willing to take the steps to make it happen. It is a libertarian concept; just as Thatcherism was going to dismantle the old monopolies and give citizens a choice of companies to provide their domestic gas or telephone services or schools, so alternativism masqueraded as another form of consumer liberation. No longer would we be tied to a single provider of health – the medical orthodoxy – but we would be free to choose. If we liked the reflexologist's eccentric view of the body as a series of energy lines which terminate in the feet, then we'd choose that; if we preferred the aromatherapist's description of the body as a collection of organs which would respond to smells, then we'd choose aromatherapy instead.

Or, as often as not, as well as rather than instead of, for one thing which many therapists had in common was their apparent ability and certain willingness to practise half a dozen or more different therapies from the same consulting room. A therapist wouldn't just be a reflexologist, but an aromatherapist, a dispenser of flower remedies and a naturopath too. And customers would happily accept this multi-skilled approach, going to their homeopath one day, their acupuncturist the next.

The temptation is to liken this to an orthodox doctor offering specialities in cardiology, oncology and gynaecology from the same consulting room, but it's not a precise comparison. All the orthodox medical specialities are based on much the same view of the body and its workings; a gynaecologist will make the same assumptions about the way the kidneys dispose of waste matter or the way the blood moves oxygen around the body as the cardiologist. The alternative practices each have subtly different views of the basis of human physiology, though; one will see it as a collection of energy lines which will respond to massage, another as a set of connected organs which will respond to infinitesimally small doses of poison. In some cases these views don't invalidate each other, in others they're mutually exclusive.

In either case, they are almost certainly wrong.

Of course I won't pretend that it wasn't gratifying to discover that my journalistic researches justified my prejudices as a consumer, but the fact remains that however hard I searched I could find little evidence for the claims made for most alternative therapies. Not that it's simply a case of saying that alternative medicine doesn't work. In fact, the failure of the therapies to come up with the goods falls into one or more of the following categories:

1 The outright sham

These are remedies that not only don't do what their promoters say they will do but which couldn't possibly do what the promoters say they will do. What sets them aside from the rest of the treatments is that the promoters know this and cynically carry on selling their phoney services. The most obvious of these is something like psychic surgery – in which various unsuspected growths are removed from the patient's interior in a procedure which involves a lot of noise and gore but, miraculously, no incision or scar – which has been shown time and time again to involve the techniques not of the psychic or the surgeon, but those of the stage magician. Given that the psychic surgeon must *know* he's palmed a small bag of ox blood and that he's spent years perfecting ways of conning people into believing that the handful of beef cartilage he produces with a flourish at the end of the 'operation' comes from the patient's innards, it's impossible to credit him with anything but the most cynical motives.

2 The impossible cure

These are treatments and diagnoses which don't and can't work, but which are usually offered in good faith by the practitioner. Often they're based on erroneous and disproven theories about the workings of the body, which predate modern medical science by some hundreds of years.

3 The improbable cure
In which category I'd place treatments which research says don't work and which common sense and a knowledge of basic scientific rules say shouldn't work, but about which there remains some fuzziness at the edge of the argument. See, for instance, homeopathy.

4 The overstated cure
There are a number of therapies which are patently capable of having some effect, but nothing like the effect promised by their most ardent promoters. There is some evidence, for instance, that osteopathy can deal with various and usually minor aches and pains, but none that it can perform the curative miracles which some claim for it.

5 The optimistic cure
Which, in fact, is a low-key version of the above. Optimistic cures are those which make the patient feel better (for which read happier, in less pain, more relaxed, more able to live with the symptoms of an illness or the side-effects of its treatment) for some time but which actually have no effect on organic illness itself.

In the years I've been researching this book – a period which includes those years when I didn't actually know I was researching this book but thought I was merely researching the many articles I've written for the press on alternative medicine – I've yet to come across much to make me change my mind about the efficacy of much alternative medicine. But then I have what alternative practitioners and their supporters will probably think is a cop-out clause, for as far as I'm concerned it's not a question of alternative medicine not working but of the classification not actually existing. There are interventions one can make which have some effect on illness and there are interventions one can make which have no effect at all. The former count as medicine, the latter don't.

Thus one of the current claims made by the alternativists is that St John's wort, for years used by herbalists as a treatment for depression, has been shown to have a real effect on that illness and that therefore this is proof that alternative medicine works. Well, yes: St John's wort has been subjected to proper clinical trials and has been shown to relieve depression. That makes it a medicine, not an alternative medicine. Inasmuch as we know how it works, it relieves depression by interacting with the brain's activity in the same way as any other antidepressant does. If it's less toxic or has fewer side-effects than synthetic antidepressants this isn't simply because it's natural: arsenic is natural too. It doesn't work because herbalists have a different view of the way the body works: the body works to its own laws not those of the observer. To say, as some therapists do, that there are many and equally valid maps of the body's workings is to say that there are many and equally valid road maps of London. There aren't: on every valid map of London the only way you can get from the Tower of London to Bermondsey is by crossing the Thames and if you try doing it any other way you're going to finish up getting very wet. (And please: no letters from smug lateral thinkers to explain how you can make the journey on dry land by going to the source of the Thames in Gloucestershire, OK?)

It's the same with the body. However much you might want to believe otherwise, the blood will still carry oxygen from the lungs to the heart; the stomach will still refuse to distinguish between salicylic acid which comes from the bark of the willow tree and that which comes from Bayer's aspirin factory; the immune system will still not respond to the non-existent amounts of active chemical in a homeopathic preparation.

Throughout the book I refer, for the most part, to 'alternative' rather than complementary medicine, which is the term alternative practitioners prefer these days. In the past, alternativists (which neologism I use to include practitioners and their customers) have accused me of a general stubbornness on the matter of alternative medicine, and said that if I were only a little more open-minded I would at least give their techniques a try. (Some go as far as to accuse me of suicidal tendencies: if, they say, I really wanted to cure my cancer then I'd try anything, however misguided I might think it to be. You'll have to trust me on this: I enjoy life, I have a wife and two small children who, I believe, want more than anything else for me to go on living. If I thought for a moment that there was a chance that Essiac or Gerson diets or any of the other remedies would make a difference then I'd try them.) In fact, as far as I'm concerned, I'm only stubborn on the matter of sticking to the old terminology, and it's for this reason.

A hundred years ago the country was full of psychics doing the most remarkable things for the delight of rooms full of believers in the paranormal. Credulous reports talk of grand pianos being hurled about, of apparitions manifesting themselves at a spiritualist's command, of gallons of ectoplasm flying around suburban living rooms. Over the years various researchers set themselves the task of testing the validity of these phenomena, and the more they researched the less impressive the phenomena became. Every time another set of pulley-strung cables was revealed holding a up grand piano, every time another projector was discovered hiding behind the curtains, so the psychics' ambitions would diminish slightly.

It's much the same with alternative medicine. When alternative therapies started coming back into vogue in the Seventies all sorts of claims were made for them: they could cure cancer, they could banish heart disease, they could deal with the most intractable illnesses. And then researchers started to test these claims, and as the research started to show that patients dosed on Laetrile died of their cancer just as quickly as those who took nothing at all, that patients who followed a strict homeopathic regimen were, all else being equal, as prone to heart disease as anyone else, so the claims began to diminish. These techniques, it turned out, weren't an *alternative* to orthodox medicine: they were *complementary* to it. You wouldn't get better by taking alternative medicine alone: no – you must take the orthodox medicine and, just to make sure it worked, the complementary medicine too.

If that sounds a touch sneering it's because I've heard the argument given a dozen different ways. As I explain in Chapter Six I've met people who swear blind they were cured of their cancer by Gerson therapy – until it turns out that they were being given therapeutic doses of radiotherapy at the same time. I know people who tell me their ulcer was absolutely cured by homeopathy – and only reveal when pressed that they were also taking antibiotics. I'm prepared to believe that there are some alternative regimes which improve the daily lot of the seriously ill patient and I don't deny that I've had a couple of massages with aromatherapy oil which made me feel rather happier when I was undergoing chemotherapy. And if that was all that alternative medicine was about – if it truly was about complementing orthodox medicine or helping customers suffering from minor but chronic illnesses lead a happier life – then I wouldn't have bothered to write this book.

But there are some major problems I have with alternative medicine as it is practised, if not by all, then by many. The first is that whenever I write about the subject I receive letters from, say, homeopaths telling me, as one such recent letter had it, that 'reputable practitioners would never claim to be able to cure cancer using homeopathy alone', which may be true, but then again it doesn't alter the fact that I've had letters from many practitioners who seem to believe themselves to be entirely reputable and who make precisely that claim. More: there are dozens of books and scores of apparently convincing websites which advise cancer sufferers not simply that orthodox treatments are still a little more hit and miss than the orthodoxy would have us believe, but that orthodox treatments simply don't work at all – that radiotherapy is more likely to cause cancer than cure it, that chemotherapy is just a fancy and expensive way of administering deadly poisons, that surgery will usually do nothing more than release stray cancer cells to wander through the body starting new and deadly colonies elsewhere.

Orthodox cancer cures are often painful and debilitating and while many cancers are treatable now, about half the time the best that's on offer is a limited prolongation of life. Who could blame a patient for being tempted by the claim that alternative therapies will do the job better, more safely and less uncomfortably – and simply skipping the orthodox stuff? It's not just cancer, either. It's not so long since a young girl died because her parents believed a naturopath's claims that he could treat her diabetes more successfully than could a doctor wielding a syringe full of insulin. Doctors in all fields regularly see the results of people treating themselves with herbs and potions which are presumed safe because they're 'natural'.

And now the alternativists are demanding ever more Health Service money both to test their claims and to implement them. As I say, I have no problem with GPs who offer their patients palliative treatments based on the massages, relaxation techniques and counselling routines around which many of the alternative therapies are built. Anything which makes the patient happier, genuinely less reliant on drugs and better equipped to deal with life is a good thing. But I worry about spending the limited amounts of money the NHS has to try to prove claims which are unprovable in order to keep the alternative lobby quiet. What follows is an argument against that lobby.

And before I start the argument proper, and before the alternativists start penning their letters complaining, as they always do, that I'm being unfair to the poor and put-upon alternative medicine industry, let me give you a simple statistic: I've just logged on to Amazon.co.uk, the Internet's largest British bookstore, and asked for a list of all the books they have on alternative medicine. The list was some 700 books long and, life being as short as it is, I asked to see the top fifty. Of them, forty-nine were books actively promoting various alternative remedies for ailments ranging from allergies and backache to heart disease, diabetes and cancer. Only one – a book published under the aegis of the American Medical Association – was anything other than absolutely in favour of alternativism.

Let's see if I can do something to correct that imbalance. After all, correcting imbalances is something that alternative medicine is usually all in favour of.

CHAPTER TWO

THIRTY YEARS OR more ago I used to wait for the bus to school each day outside a small, dark and forbidding shop at Dalston Junction in east London. The shop may well have had its proprietor's name over the door, but all I can remember were the words painted in flaking gold leaf on the sill beneath the dusty window, which read 'Surgical Supplies'. In the days before high-street chemists had bright and tempting dump-bins next to the till, full of the latest in multi-ribbed, extra-stimulating, sundried-tomato-flavoured condoms, every neighbourhood had a shop like this. The gloomy window displays were all much the same: there would be a too-pink plaster representation of the human leg from lower thigh to shin with, wrapped around its knee, a patent bandage for relieving joint pain; there would be a contraption made of canvas, leather and rubber which turned out to be a truss for hernia sufferers (I say 'turned out' because in this still-decorous era it would never be labelled as such); there would be a small, red, neon sign at the front of the display reading, simply, 'Durex'; and there would be a couple of adverts for patent medicines which weren't available on the National Health. The one I remember best was Tiger Balm, an ointment which you rubbed on to relieve any number of aches and sprains and which even in the mid-Sixties seemed to me to be hopelessly old-fashioned.

(And just to show how little I know: I've just looked up Tiger Balm on the Internet, partly out of nostalgia and partly on the off chance that one of those nerdish sites which fondly lists the history of Olde English Flavoured Spangles and Aztec Bars would have more details about the embrocation than I could remember, and guess what? Not only is Tiger Balm still made in Tunbridge Wells from a mixture of 'camphor, menthol, cajuput oil and clove oil. It contains no animal products', but it has its own website – *http://www.tigerbalm.co.uk/*.)

And in the middle of all this was a smaller, more discreet sign reading 'Herbal Remedies'. Thirty years ago this was still the place for herbalism, which, if it was considered at all, was as an esoteric practice left over from a previous age, an age which stretched from the early twentieth century back to the Middle Ages and before. It was an age when orthodox medicine was expensive, even more limited in its abilities than it is now, and altogether something of a hit-and-miss affair. Indeed, for much of the time the overlap between the orthodoxy, defined by its members having passed the standard medical and surgical exams and being members of the various professional bodies, and traditional medicine – as it was usually called in those days – was pretty substantial. As a child I remember our GP, one Dr Soldinger, prescribing something called Black Ointment for almost every minor ailment, and a couple of the major ones too. Pharmacists seemed able enough to dispense the prescription then although I can find no mention of it in the current *British National Formulary* and have no idea what the stuff was. But certainly there was the sense that this was not so much a modern doctor handing out treatments carefully tailored to individuals and their illnesses, but rather a local shaman in a rumpled suit with access to a specific herbal panacea, which he would offer in much the same way as a couple of centuries earlier the local wise man might have offered powdered orris root.

But by the time I started waiting each day for the bus outside the surgical supplies shop, all that had changed. Its herbal remedies were the products of what was seen as a quaint medical backwater. In the past few decades – and especially in response to a war which had finished just twenty years earlier – medicine had made the sort of massive breakthroughs which allowed its practitioners and patients to believe that nothing was impossible.

In 1930, for instance, the US had 600 tuberculosis sanatoriums with 84,000 beds between them and some 175 Americans in every 100,000 were dying of the disease. By the mid-Sixties the discovery and introduction of antibiotics had slashed that figure to about two per 100,000 and until the disease started to fight back in the late Eighties and early Nineties, the figure dropped further still to about one in 100,000, turning it from a disease which struck often and at random into a medical curiosity which one was more likely to come across in the history books than in the local hospital.

Other major diseases were being defeated too. Between them, mass immunisation programmes and novel medical treatments had seen off, or soon would, diphtheria, smallpox and whooping cough. Some days at the same bus stop at which I queued I'd seen an elderly man with no nose; he was, local rumour had it, a tertiary syphilitic, his missing nose a sign of God's compassion, John Donne had written some hundreds of years earlier, which prevented such sinners smelling their own rotting flesh. But he was a rarity: syphilis and the other sexually transmitted diseases were conquerable too. (At this point, of course, nobody had heard about AIDS.)

These were, it can hardly be disputed, successes for orthodox medicine. You may believe that there are alternative remedies which can deal with TB or diphtheria or syphilis, and I'm happy to allow you to cling to that belief for the time being at least, but the reason the number of TB sufferers diminished over that period was because of the discovery of antibiotics, their testing under laboratory conditions and their ready availability. Whether homeopathy or herbalism could have done the job doesn't matter, because the fact is that they didn't.

There were still major killers abroad, of course, in particular cancer and heart disease. But we knew that it wouldn't be long before we would find cures for these as well. Already cancer sufferers were three times as likely to survive for five years after diagnosis than they'd been at the turn of the century, and who could not believe that any year now the cure for all cancers would be discovered? In 1967 Christiaan Barnard had just performed the first heart transplant in South Africa, and even if his was a reckless operation doomed to failure we knew that eventually it would become as routine a procedure as bypass surgery was, indeed, about to be.

It seemed that there was no part of our lives which the new medicine wasn't prepared to deal with. Maternity hospitals in the Sixties were happily trying to turn the process of child-birth into something painless and timetabled, with new techniques for inducing birth during office hours so it didn't interfere with the consultant's golf arrangements; schools marshalled their children into lines to receive free spectacles and dental fillings and sugar lumps doped with magical immunising fluids. New drugs were being developed which could control our appetites, our weight, our moods.

The time would come, next year, or the year after, or the year after that, when we would all live happily and healthily and die of old age somewhere in our early eighties. We didn't need herbal remedies from dark, dank shops, where we'd have to mingle with shame-faced customers in for their nasty ointments and their disgusting surgical appliances. Had we come this far just so that we could treat ourselves with Tiger Balm?

But were we impressed by the prospect of our new longevity, our promised happy, healthiness? Not a bit of it. For all the old geezers we meet in the pub whose philosophy on life is summed up by the rubric 'Well, as long as you've got your health, is what I always say . . .', the fact is that health is something we usually appreciate only when it's not there. Our fore-bears, in the age of un-health, didn't live as long as we did, but nor did they expect to. They took it for granted that life was a condition beset by arbitrary and inexplicable aches and pains and growths and the various pustulant evidences of bodily decay. There were, to be sure, those professionals and edu-cated amateurs who could suggest some remedy or another, but if the remedies didn't work that was as much the fault of the illness itself as it was of the doctor or the herbalist.

But we expected more. Hell, we'd been *promised* more. Just as we'd learned, rightly, to expect that the political system could be arranged to provide a roof over the head and food in the stomach of all of us, so, we believed, could the medical system be arranged to give us all health and happiness. It was our *right*, dammit.

And the medical establishment, flattered by all those pieces in the popular press describing the latest miracle cure which was just about – always just about – to arrive at the local surgery, joined in with the celebrations and connived with the scam. Indeed, if the boom in alternative medicine is anybody's fault it's that of orthodox medicine. It was the orthodoxy – helped by the media and our own vanity – which allowed us to believe that we could all be healthy and happy, that there was a pill for every problem and that if we died too early or too painfully it was an act of some agency other than capricious old God. The orthodoxy allowed us to expect miracles and then, when it couldn't provide them, got annoyed when we started looking elsewhere.

And the elsewhere we looked to was the alternative practitioners. They were only too willing to take our custom and if the orthodox practitioners were willing to let us believe in medical miracles then the alternativists were doubly so.

And the alternativists had one massive advantage working in their favour: most of us have not the faintest idea how medicine works.

Come to that, most of us have a pretty feeble idea of how our body works. What percentage of the population do you think knows what a busy spleen does for its living, or a pancreas or a liver? A recent episode of the BBC's game show *The Generation Game* asked contestants to place stickers naming various bones and organs on the bodies of a couple of bathing-suited models. Both teams of bright, ordinary citizens who looked as though they might have some basic biology at school scored a fat zero. Look at any advert for those cosmetics which claim to rid the body of 'toxins' and you'll understand what the popular understanding of the function of the kidneys is. Then look at the ads for moisturisers, which claim somehow to be able to deliver beneficial water through the skin and you'll understand how few consumers have worked out that if water molecules were small enough to penetrate our body coverings we'd dissolve in the first shower of rain like the Wicked Witch of the West in *The Wizard of Oz*.

How many of us have any idea what happens when we treat a headache with aspirin? When a hard-pressed doctor hands out yet another prescription for an antibiotic in the full knowledge that it can have no possible effect on the virus the patient has dragged into the surgery with him, he does so because it's easier to give a prescription-demanding patient ('Well, the *other* doctor always gives me one . . .') something than to explain why nothing would do the job just as well.

Don't get me wrong: I'm not saying that we should all be amateur doctors able to argue the case for amoxycillin against that of tetracycline with our GPs. After all, the reason we demand that professional doctors train for so long and have to pass such difficult tests before they're allowed to practise is because most of us don't have the time, ability or inclination to do the job ourselves.

But the absence of even the most basic understanding of the workings of the body and the laws which govern those workings not only allows for lazy and inept orthodox doctors, but allows thousands of alternative practitioners to make claims which to most of us seem just as reasonable as the claims made by the orthodoxy. After all, if we accept that a basic principle of orthodox medicine is that a pill will somehow make a headache or a rash or a pain disappear, why cannot that same basic principle apply to homeopathy or herbalism or naturopathy? If a doctor is telling the truth when he says that penicillin will make the blotches on our stomach disappear then why should we assume that a herbalist is telling a lie when he says that a Bach flower remedy will make those same blotches go away? If we have no sense of the causal relationship between ailment and symptom or between treatment and cure, how can we be expected to differentiate between legitimate treatments and illegitimate ones?

Especially given that, for all its promises, orthodox medicine proved itself patently incapable of dealing with the illnesses which beset us most of the time. It's no good claiming that while our grandparents had only a 20 per cent chance of surviving cancer, modern therapies mean that in parts of Europe and the US a cancer patient now has a 50 per cent chance of surviving for five years – when what we most often see is the 50 per cent who don't survive. (In fact the survival rate in Britain is slightly over 40 per cent – another failure for orthodox medicine.) Yes, our hearts are susceptible to all sorts of invasive treatments when they go wrong, but keeping them from going wrong seems to mean living the sort of Spartan life which is in direct contradiction to the lotus-eating life promised us at the same time we were being promised universal health.

And in any case, these are just the illnesses which most regularly shove us, sweating, up against the crash-barriered entrances to the local hospital. When modern man says he's ill what he more usually means is that he has the sort of illness which affects not his heart or his cellular make-up, but his temperament, his muscles, his concentration. They are what his medieval relatives would have described as diseases of his humours – he feels too melancholy or bilious or not sanguine or phlegmatic enough. All too often his diseases are, in the etymological sense of the word, just that: dis-eases.

For a while orthodox medicine thought it had even those vague and non-specific illnesses licked, and for a glorious few years in the late Sixties and early Seventies GPs would happily dole out Valium and its variants in the benzodiazepine group to anyone who turned up wanting no more than for life to be a little more bearable. And when it emerged that Valium was addictive, stopped working after a while and turned vital but anxious patients into blank-faced zombies, even that was no longer any sort of real recourse. It meant that when Prozac turned up a few years later, together with a gleeful chorus of (mainly American) doctors claiming that it could make us all happy all the time, we were less prepared to believe that the orthodox magic would work.

But we could still believe in the non-orthodox magic, because we still believed that there must be some magic somewhere to believe in. And while we'd learned that orthodox medicine was not only fallible but could also be dangerous, addictive or even merely debilitating, the one thing we knew about alternative medicine was that it was safe. It was 'natural'.

There are, of course, a number of problems with this, the most obvious being that 'natural' is by no means a synonym for 'safe'. I have in the garden aconite, digitalis and euphorbia: all are used in various alternative (and orthodox) therapies and while the milky sap of euphorbia will merely burn the skin, a small amount of the first two will kill. What, after all, do you think the hemlock which killed Socrates was, if not the entirely natural and very pretty little relative of the carrot? Even 'natural' remedies which are happily sold over the counter can be highly toxic and an overdose of, say, feverfew – an anti-inflammatory prescribed by herbalists where an orthodox doctor might suggest a couple of aspirin – can have nasty side-effects.

But, fair enough: not even the most ardent alternativist would argue with the toxic possibilities of mother nature. Indeed, many of them rather like the deistic idea of nature as both compassionate saviour as well as a fierce enemy when not given its due respect. The problem comes when they try to distinguish between two identical substances, one grown in nature's rich earth and the other synthesised in the inhuman and sterile lab. Willow bark, for instance, has been used for centuries as an antipyretic, anti-inflammatory and mild painkiller. It's been used, indeed, in much the same way as we'd use aspirin. Which is hardly surprising, given that as long ago as 1838 chemists identified the active ingredient of willow bark as salicylic acid – from *salix*, the botanical name for the willow family – of which one synthesised form is acetylsalicylic acid, better known as aspirin. If you were to take a tablet of pure, natural salicylic acid derived from a willow tree and a tablet of nasty scientific salicylic acid which had popped out of a stainless steel tube at the Bayer factory, it would be impossible to tell the difference between them by any means known to man. Both consist of the same subatomic particles making up identical atoms which are clustered together in identical ways to form identical molecules. A chemist couldn't tell the difference and a herbalist couldn't tell the difference. Come to that, not even a herbalist who believes there *is* a difference could tell the difference.

More to the point, your body couldn't tell the difference: both pills would have precisely the same chemical reaction with the pain receptors in your brain, with the delicate lining of your stomach. At this level 'natural' is meaningless. As, of

25

course is the nature-lovers' other favourite demon word, 'chemical'. Read the packages of some 'natural' products – remedies, supplements, foods – and you'll often come across the claim that the product contains 'no chemical additives' or even – albeit rarely these days – 'no chemicals'. Which means what, precisely? The word 'chemical' doesn't describe only those substances which are found in laboratories or synthesised in factories. Our body is made entirely of chemicals; so is every substance, however mud-covered and dewily natural, in the herbalist's manual. Come to that, mud and dew are composed of chemicals.

But this is piffling stuff with which few alternativists would argue. My point, though, is not that there is any debate about the meaning of 'natural' or 'chemical' among those who have even the most basic understanding of the natural sciences, but that these terms are used to promote remedies, as if they conferred upon them some special powers. It's perhaps unfortunate that the word 'natural' has two allied meanings; it describes something which occurs in nature and also something which feels right, comfortable, legitimate. Anything which doesn't occur in nature is, by that definition at least, 'unnatural', which itself is a synonym for wrong or abhorrent.

It's this very idea of 'naturalness' which is the basis for so many misconceptions about what alternative medicine is, what it does, and how it works. It's an idea which leads to conclusions varying from the odd to the laughable. 'Natural' medicine, we are told, for instance, is used successfully by those ancient cultures which have a greater sense of the bond between man and his environment than alienated Western man does these days. Really? It's easy for the well-fed metropolitan with time and money on his hands to talk about dealing with his chronic symptoms with ayurvedic medicine or Chinese herbal therapies, or ancient African or Native American remedies, but if you go to the countries where those remedies are all they have, you'll find them crying out for good old Western antibiotics, painkillers and all the rest of the modern and expensive pharmacopoeia. A Ugandan dying of AIDS-related tuberculosis doesn't want to be treated with the natural remedies of his forefathers: he wants an aseptic syringe full of antibiotics and then he wants to join the sixteen-pill-a-day programme which, in the West, would stand a chance of putting his AIDS on hold. When the government of South Africa complains that not enough is being done to help the 10 per cent of its population which is HIV-positive it isn't asking for help with preparing 'natural' remedies: it wants AZT.

Even in those countries where traditional remedies are thought of as preponderant and successful the move is towards Western treatments. In China there is now a massive discrepancy between the health of those who live in the cities and use, for the most part, Western medicine and rural dwellers who use traditional remedies. Yes: city dwellers tend to be better off, and better-off people tend to be healthier, but the fact remains that for all the burgeoning number of Chinese health clinics in the West, in China the Chinese, given the choice, will usually go for Western medicine. Who can blame them? Western medicine is based on the very scientific principles which the Chinese medical authorities are trying to apply to the local product. Fair enough: it's always difficult to determine the precise reasoning behind the actions of monolithic and morally dubious institutions such as the Chinese government, but there's no reason to suspect that when that government passes laws against con-artists masquerading as Qigong masters who are going round the countryside poisoning the peasants and charging them for the privilege, there's not a real problem here to deal with.

Meanwhile in Hong Kong one survey demonstrates that a mere 14 per cent of young people consider visiting a traditional healer with their medical problems, and in Japan, where the population has access to both traditional and modern methods, even greater numbers use the latter. In mainland China itself no more than 18 per cent of the population use traditional medicines these days, and this in a country where those therapies are cheap and available to everyone. Look at any Eastern country where traditional medicine is the medicine of choice (however unwilling that choice may be) and you'll find a country with high infant mortality, a country where people die young, where illnesses and disease we treat routinely with easily available drugs cause pain and suffering. Traditional remedies are wonderful if you live in the West and need to deal with nothing more pressing than the odd rash, irritable bowel or anxiety attack and if you have a modern pharmacopoeia to fall back on if things get difficult; they're useless against the diseases which daily kill and maim the inhabitants of the countries from where those remedies come.

So why do so many of us say we prefer the natural to the scientific?

I am not an academic and this is not an academic book, even though the facts I list in it have a perfectly good scientific basis to them. But when it comes to human motivation I'm working blind. I can only guess why most people seem to prefer the unproven to the proven, the anecdotal to the rigorously demonstrated, the so-called natural to the scientific. And the guess I make is a journalistic one: 'natural' makes for a better story.

We are living in the second great age of anti-intellectualism. The first lasted all the way from the disappearance of the ancient Greeks and slightly less ancient Romans with their early, if shaky, reliance on observation, logic and scientific proof, to the coming of the Enlightenment. That particular anti-intellectualism came as a result of our not knowing enough. The world was a complicated place and man didn't have enough information to explain it in any other than irrational terms. The irrationalism led to religious and political dogma and that in turn led to the suppression of those who would try to explain the universe in ways which didn't involve the cupidity of gods and angels.

The new anti-intellectualism comes about, I think, because we know too much. As a child in the Fifties there was still, just about, a sense that a bright and well-educated person could get a handle on most of the things that made the world work. A basic knowledge of the natural sciences would be enough to explain most of what we saw about us: the wonders of radio, television, medicine, architecture, industrial techniques and so on. At the age of eight I took two magazines each week: the old-fashioned and about-to-fold *Children's Newspaper*, founded by Arthur Mee of the *Children's Encyclopaedia*, and

28

the glossy new *Look and Learn*. Each week these papers would be filled with colourful articles explaining how things worked and there was little in the world which couldn't be reduced to the sort of fact that an eight-year-old could understand.

It wasn't just children who could keep on top of things. A general practitioner could keep up with medical science pretty well with a subscription to the *Lancet*, and an engineer by reading whatever journal engineers had in the Fifties. Cars were still built in such a way that most drivers with a few basic skills could keep them going and for most of us 'technology' meant the phone, the radio, the TV set and a few consumer electrical bits and pieces in the kitchen. Changes, when they came, seemed to be in giant leaps: the sort of thing the press could describe as 'miracles'. We lived in an age when we would go to bed in a world without swipe cards or portable phones or home computers and wake up in one where one or other of these things were suddenly possible.

No longer. The world in the new millennium is unknowable. There are too many facts, too many figures, too many people. Where once we were all generalists, now it is a world of specialists. Technology comes with 'no user-serviceable parts inside' stickers over everything and we have to defer to others if we want anything installed, serviced, mended, explained. *Look and Learn* went under when new science stopped being explicable in sequences of cartoon drawings. We don't understand it because we cannot understand it because there is too much of it and it's too complicated. And generally speaking that which we don't understand we fear or despise.

But at least the new technology works. Yes, we complain about computers sending us electricity bills for minus a half-penny and how we can't set the video to record *EastEnders*, and the developed world is still full of people who regard the Internet with the same suspicion as our bumpkin forebears once regarded the telephone. But generally we understand that the technological novelties are our servants, albeit often chippy and disrespectful servants. More, we understand that so long as it works we don't really have to understand it. If the beyond-home-servicing car goes wrong we send it to the garage; if the phone stops working we call out the phone company or, consumerism being what it is, just buy another phone for £4.95.

But the new medicine is something else. It has all the attributes of the new technology – complicated science, high cost, long-term development – but it doesn't work. Or at least it doesn't work as well as the rest of the new science. There are too few medical equivalents of the fax machine or the desktop computer, devices which, for all their impenetrability, usually work when we switch them on. Often medicine doesn't work, or doesn't work as perfectly as we'd like. It has nasty side-effects or works only for a short while or sometimes doesn't work at all. It betrays our trust in it: every time we think we have TB licked it comes back in a new form and licks us right back again.

Of course, our attitude isn't helped by the fact that we forget what life was like before the coming of the new medicine – and, again, I'm referring to medicine as it's practised only in rich and developed nations. I have a friend who, tearful and depressed, was put on a course of Prozac. She stopped being tearful and depressed and, reasonably enough, decided to come off the Prozac. At which point, of course, she became tearful and depressed again. Except that, forgetting what she was like before she started taking the drug, she blamed her current depression on the drug itself. It was because she had taken it she was tearful and depressed. It's a reasonable analogy for our attitude towards modern scientific medicine. Look at any popular newspaper piece on the apparent dangers of certain childhood immunisation regimes, or antibiotics or surgical routines, and you'd imagine that these new techniques were themselves responsible for more illness than they cure or prevent – an impression which is hardly helped by the alternativists' weasel ways with the figures for iatrogenic (i.e. medically caused) illness. The fact is, of course, that in part thanks to modern medical methods we are healthier, in less pain and longer-lived than any generation which preceded us.

But, as I say, medicine is an imperfect science. And, worse, we don't seem to be bright enough to understand the reasons for its imperfection. When things go wrong we find ourselves hostage to men and women who use language we don't understand, talk of scientific principles we don't have the learning to grasp, who seem to be more confident than their results would allow, who offer us treatments which seem to work on some random basis which is never explained to us.

No wonder so many of us take the easy way out. Alternative medicine makes none of the demands of us that scientific medicine makes. When an iridologist tells us the story of the discovery of his science it's one we can understand only too easily. It reads like a fairy story: boy finds owl with broken leg; owl has big spot in his iris; boy heals broken leg, spot goes away; boy goes on to discover that by studying spots in the iris he can diagnose all illnesses. What's not to understand? When we read about how Dr Bach discovered his flower remedies it makes perfect sense on a sort of flowers-are-harbingers-of-good level which wouldn't have grasped the public imagination quite so forcefully, I imagine, if he'd used thirty-eight types of spider to produce the Bach spider remedies.

In journalistic terms 'natural' is certainly the better story. Alternativism provides us with the continual stream of stories which we've come to expect. Real scientific progress is slow and boring and provides tiny changes: newspapers can't run 'cancer: still no cure' stories that often, but there are always plenty of alternative therapy stories for them to run – if not as news stories, then at least in the back pages in the 'You and Your Health' sections.

Not only is alternativism a better provider of stories, but the stories are the ones the press like best. They're stories of the little guy against the monolithic forces of science or money; it's the with-one-bound-he-was-free story rewritten in medical terms. It's a story of that which science never respects: natural justice. In the alternative world people don't recover because they put their faith in Glaxo or Pfizer or Upjohn, but because they put their faith in flowers or the wisdom of the ancients. The alternative world is one where the people who live are the ones who really *want* to live, which is to say – according to the pure principles of natural justice – the ones who deserve to live.

Here's an example.

A few months ago one of my readers, irritated rather than outraged by my continual mounting of my anti-alternativism hobby horse, sent me by way of rebuttal a story from his local paper in Brighton. It was of a man with cancer for whom the local hospital could do, said the paper, nothing more. But the man, not willing to take such a grim prognosis lying down, had learned of a foreign clinic which was regularly curing cancers such as his. He had raised some £20,000 from local well-wishers to pay for his treatment. It was a cheery story and never mind that the clinic he was flying off to had as much chance of curing him of his cancer as did the local chiropodist. Nobody at the paper had thought to ask his doctors what they thought of the trip or even why a relatively poor and backward country was apparently able to offer a cure, where Britain – a country which spends four times as much of a much higher GDP on health – wasn't. Nor does the paper seemed to have checked with one of the dozens of resources which would have told them that the clinic was staffed by quacks using a technique which had been roundly demonstrated as bogus any number of times. For who wants to read a story headlined 'Local Man Suckered by Con-Artists: Will Die Soon' when they could have a story reading 'Plucky Brighton Man Raises £20,000 for Miracle Cancer Cure'?

Does the story do any harm? On its own, probably not: we've always liked reading stories about miracles because they buttress the belief, I suppose, that a miracle might come into our own lives one day. But stories like this also add to the constant drip, drip, drip which undermines our faith in real medicine, in real science, in the techniques which haven't brought a cure to all cancer patients but have brought help to many of them, which have wiped out so many once-fatal diseases, which have provided what twenty or a hundred years ago really would have been regarded as miracles. Which itself might not matter were it not that our health is such big business and is run to a large extent by politicians who react to consumer-led voting rather than to rational debate. In the US it's precisely this sort of story which has led to the formation of the Office of Alternative Medicine under the aegis of Senator Tom Harkin, a man who has championed the cause of various therapies many of which are at best unproven.

Perhaps that faith needs undermining, of course, but telling fairy stories about miracle workers isn't the way to go about it.

CHAPTER THREE

I'LL COME CLEAN. I am an alternative practitioner myself, after a fashion. There: I've said it.

I have a four-year-old son who, as is the way with four-year-old sons, climbs on things and then falls off them, losing chunks of skin and blood on the way down to the ground. And whenever this happens – about four times a week on average – and he runs to me, crying and pointing to the latest graze, I apply strictly alternative remedies. I don't give him strong drugs to kill the pain or staunch the flow of blood but I clean the tiny wound, ask him what happened, sympathise with him about the fickleness of gravity and the harshness of brick, sit him on my lap with a glass of water, kiss him and rub the hurt better. And it works, every time.

So what do you think I should call the technique? Fatheratherapy? Dynamic parentesiology? Because dealing with minor problems by calm talking, sitting down quietly and rubbing it better seems to be just what much alternative therapy is all about.

Take a look at any of the tables which show how regularly the citizens in developed countries now use alternative therapies. There are equivalent figures for all the developed countries, and although they vary proportionately in the types of remedy used – France is heavy on homeopathy, for instance, and Germany on herbalism – they all show that anything between a third and a half of us use or have used such remedies in any given twelve-month period, a figure which is used by the alternativists to show how popular they are (with the implication that popularity equals effectiveness) and by the various medical associations and schools to justify spending precious funds on appeasing the alternative lobby. Impressive as the figures are, they're pretty meaningless in terms of what they tell us about alternative users.

If you've been paying attention you'll have gathered by now that my own answer to the question 'Do you use alternative medicine?' would be a simple 'No'. But then in statistical terms that's not quite true. Like most people I sometimes have trouble sleeping. If I take a prescribed sleeping pill – temazepam, say – then I know I'll feel pretty groggy in the morning. And so from time to time I've used a commercial preparation of the herb valerian to help me sleep. Valerian works well enough as a fairly gentle soporific for perfectly good biochemical reasons,* but my occasional use of it doesn't mean I'm about to subject my corns or my tumours to the ministrations of a herbalist. Nonetheless, I would count as an alternative medicine user in these statistics, just as much as would the man visiting his homeopath three times a week.

So let's try to break some of these statistics down. One of the most comprehensive US studies demonstrates the growth in alternative use over the years from 1990 to 1997. The figures for 1997 are shown in Table 1.

Let's imagine, for a moment, that we've never come across the term 'alternative medicine' and try to extract from this table something rather more useful than raw statistics.

You don't have to be too much of a cynic to translate the first entry in the list and the most popular use of alternative therapy – going to a masseuse or an osteopath** with a back problem – as 'When I have a sore back, I get somebody who

---

* Since you ask, the active ingredient in valerian root has an affinity for GABA receptors, GABA – gamma-amniobutyric acid – being a non-essential amino acid that functions as a neurotransmitter in the central nervous system by decreasing neuron activity.

** Osteopathy and chiropractic are not, I realise, strictly the same. But in the US – whence comes this research – chiropractors are used by those who in Britain would usually use osteopaths.

Condition	% reporting condition	% who used alternative therapy for condition in last twelve months	% who saw alternative practitioner for condition in last twelve months	% who both saw medical doctor and used alternative therapy in last twelve months	% who saw both medical doctor and alternative practitioner for condition in last twelve months	Therapies most commonly used for condition
Back problems	24.0	47.6	30.1	58.8	39.1	Chiropractic, massage
Allergies	20.7	16.6	4.2	28.0	6.4	Herbalism, relaxation
Fatigue	16.7	27.0	6.3	51.6	13.1	Relaxation, massage
Arthritis	16.6	26.7	10.0	38.5	15.9	Relaxation, chiropractic
Headaches	12.9	32.2	13.3	42.0	20.0	Relaxation, chiropractic
Neck problems	12.1	57.0	37.5	66.6	47.5	Chiropractic, massage
High blood pressure	10.9	11.7	0.9	11.9	1.1	Mega-vitamins, relaxation
Sprains or strains	10.8	23.6	10.3	29.4	15.9	Chiropractic, relaxation
Insomnia	9.3	26.4	7.6	48.4	13.3	Relaxation, herbalism
Lung problems	8.7	13.2	2.5	17.9	3.4	Relaxation, spiritual healing, herbalism
Skin problems	8.6	6.7	2.2	6.8	0.0	Imagery, energy healing
Digestive problems	8.2	27.3	9.7	34.1	10.7	Relaxation, herbalism
Depression	5.6	40.9	15.6	40.9	26.9	Relaxation, spiritual healing
Anxiety	5.5	42.7	11.6	42.7	21.0	Relaxation, spiritual healing

Table 1   Use of alternative medicine in US, 1997[*]

[*] Taken from D.M. Eisenberg, R.B. Davis, S.L. Ettner, S. Appel, S. Wilkey, M. Van Rompay and R.C. Kessler, 'Trends in Alternative Medicine Use in the United States 1990–1997', *Journal of the American Medical Association* (11 November 1998), pp. 1569–75.

knows what they're doing to rub it better.' Or there's the third most popular treatment: relaxation and massage used to treat fatigue. In the non-alternative world that becomes the tediously prosaic 'When I'm tired I lie down.' Much the same goes for headaches and relaxation, which become 'When I've been working too hard it helps if I lie down in a darkened room for a bit' or anxiety – 'Anxious? Just lie down and think calming thoughts for a while.'

Don't get me wrong: I'm not sneering. I accept, from personal experience as much as anything else, that conditions such as chronic backache, inexplicable fatigue, too-frequent headaches, are real and debilitating. But I also accept that the formalised and refined equivalents of 'rubbing it better' really do work for many of the problems we all get from time to time; talking calmly to somebody who loves us (which is how my son sees it) or to somebody who will listen with understanding, patience and respect (which is how one might describe an alternative therapist) will obviously have an effect on how we perceive our symptoms. It's interesting, for instance, that over sixty years after the NHS started, so many people still prefer to pay to see a private GP. Whatever the faults of the NHS, and they are many and substantial, few complain that they can't actually get to see their GP or that having got to see him or her they can't get advice or treatment of some sort or another. So why pay when you can get it for free? Because while a GP who sees you on the NHS is unlikely to give you more than ten minutes of their time – and six is the national average for what is laughably still called a consultation – a doctor who gets to submit his invoice for professional services rendered is unlikely to strangle that particular golden-egg-laying goose by giving his patients anything other than time and understanding. Go to an NHS GP with the vague symptoms that take up so much of his working day and as often as not you'll be given pretty short shrift: even if he wanted to determine the reasons behind the recurring headaches or the continual tiredness, he wouldn't have the time to do so without breaking his contract with the local health authority to give all his patients a little time rather than some of them a lot.

Which is where alternative medicine does so well. On average an alternative therapist will spend over an hour with a patient on a first visit and at least half an hour on subsequent visits. The hour will be spent in a room designed to calm and relax, and, as with a private GP, the questions will be respectful, there will be no suggestion that your complaint is imagined or too footling to deal with, or that your response to the condition is inappropriate to its severity. It's like talking to a wise friend, except that the therapist will, at all times, talk about *you*. Unlike your friends he will ask how *you* are without expecting you to ask about him in return. He will listen to your problems without telling you all about his. Which of us is so self-effacing, so modest, so completely lacking in vanity that we wouldn't feel better, reassured, more confident after an hour of that? Add to it some gentle rubbing, some pleasant-smelling oils, some interesting homeopathic or herbal preparations made up just for *you*, for your own, personal, unique illness – and which of us doesn't want confirmation of our specialness, our uniqueness? – and the £60, or whatever it is the session costs, becomes a bargain.

And if that were all there was to alternative medicine this book would be called *Finding Your Inner Joy – Alternative Medicine for a Better You* and would be on sale in health-food shops next to the St John's wort and the ginseng.

There is no doubt that some people with some conditions do feel better some of the time if they use certain alternative therapies. Equally, there's little doubt that those orthodox medical practices where patients also have access to relaxation therapy, the various massage regimes and the talking therapies have happier patients than the practices which merely dispense prescriptions and hospital referrals. Although there are doctors who were trained in the methods of the orthodoxy and who have subsequently become fully-fledged alternativists, when the British Medical Association talks about the substantial number of practices offering these therapies on the Health Service, it's these minor therapies they're talking about.

It makes sense. An orthodox doctor is expensive to train and even more expensive to employ. Asking doctors to spend their days talking, relaxing, massaging – rubbing it better, if you like – isn't a particularly efficient way of using Health Service resources. And just as the NHS will use district nurses and in-practice nurse practitioners to give routine treatments, apply bandages, change dressings, give injections, it makes sense to use specialists in relaxation or massage to deal with minor but chronic complaints.

But to say this is not to say that, when it comes to organic disease or disruption, alternative medicine is any sort of true alternative to scientific medicine.

Most of the conditions which seem to respond to alternative therapies, for instance, are those with symptoms which can only be assessed in subjective terms. If I am discovered to have a cancer, or a heart condition or a diseased liver, then the extent and severity of the condition itself can be pretty accurately measured: the tumour is this big, the heart is beating in this particular arrhythmic pattern, the liver is working at this per cent of its full capacity. But not all illnesses – or symptoms of illnesses – can be so easily quantified.

Pain, for instance, is notoriously difficult to quantify, not only because one patient's slight ache is another's hellish agony but because individual assessment of pain varies from time to time and hour to hour. My own cancer treatment, for example, has left me with a degree of pain on the right side of my face where the jaw hinges. Sometimes, if I'm engrossed in my work or if I've had a couple of drinks, or if I'm watching a particularly enjoyable TV show, I'm hardly aware of any pain at all. As I write, for instance, I realise that I've gone for half a day without any sort of pain relief. But there are times when I'm bored, or anxious or restless in bed, when the pain feels unbearable and when I shuffle to the bathroom to dose myself with as many industrial-strength painkillers as I can find.

How do I assess that sort of pain? Is it the same quality and quantity of pain both times but I'm experiencing it differently? In purely biochemical terms are the same number of pain receptors being triggered in both circumstances, but for some reason my awareness of the pain is greater when there's less emotional background noise? Is my reaction to pain different from somebody's who hasn't been through the eight operations I've had in the past few years?

And just as it's difficult to quantify pain, and thus the relief afforded from it, so there are any number of other conditions whose severity is a matter of entirely subjective assessment. If an asthmatic is anxious, is his breathlessness objectively greater or does it just *feel* greater? Does a hay-fever sufferer feel worse in hot weather because the weather actually increases the severity of the symptoms or because equivalent symptoms feel more oppressive under the debilitating effects of a hot sun? Note that I'm not saying that experiencing a condition as more insufferable is any different from it *being* more insufferable: in metaphysical terms, at least, our senses don't lie to us and if, for whatever reason, our brain is assessing pain or breathlessness or nausea or tiredness as at level x then that's the level at which we experience it. The sentence 'You've not lost as much blood as the mess on the floor would suggest' is a legitimate one; the sentence 'It isn't hurting you as much as you think it is' isn't.

You don't even have to go into the realms of illness to find this sort of subjective reaction. Anyone who has taken even the occasional alcoholic drink knows that sometimes a glass of wine has no effect at all and sometimes that same glass will make you feel as abandoned as Oliver Reed after his first bottle or two of vodka. Do people who regularly get drunk on a small sherry do so because they are particularly susceptible to booze or because being in a boozing situation is in some way psychologically liberating? And if, driving back from the pub feeling drunk on a couple of whiskies, they suddenly see a blue light flashing in their rear-view mirror and feel immediately sober, who is to say that the sobriety is any more unreal than their intoxication? Of course, with drunkenness it is possible to quantify the effects of the booze objectively as well as subjectively: the amount of alcohol in the blood can be measured precisely, the effect on the autonomic nervous system determined, the ability of a drunk to drive a car or walk in a straight line assessed. And yet we've all met those who honestly believe they can drive better after a couple of drinks (subjective assessment) while even the most basic tests (objective assessment) will prove the opposite.

It is, in medical terms at least, a can of worms.

And expectation of the two systems of treatment make it more difficult still. Imagine: a patient turns up at his GP's surgery complaining of recurrent headaches and persistent tiredness. The doctor does the standard tests, asks the usual questions, tells the patient that he can find no disease and that he's probably working too hard. He should relax a little, cut down on some of the excesses, take aspirin for the headache. Has the doctor done his job? Well, yes, as far as he can. Will the patient think that the doctor's done his job? Probably not. He's not discovered any illness, not prescribed any drugs, not suggested any but the vaguest tactics for dealing with the problem.

On the advice of a friend the same patient goes to an alternative therapist and presents him with precisely the same symptoms. The therapist listens and doesn't get impatient when the patient tells him about his marriage, his work, his bowel movements, what he had for breakfast. He'll ask questions – not just 'How often do you get these headaches?' but something more specific and detailed: What time of day do you get them? Do they increase in severity if you eat such-and-such or drink so-and-so? He will make an assessment not of the nature of the symptoms but of the patient's whole way of life: the sort of assessment that he'll describe as 'holistic' because, he says, he treats the whole person and not just a set of symptoms.

And at the end of the consultation, and based on its revelations, the therapist will act. He'll recommend something he'll call 'a change in lifestyle', that the patient drinks less, cuts down on tea and coffee. He might offer him a cassette tape on which a calm voice will guide the patient through an hour of relaxation or a massage or some herbal or homeopathic or naturopathic remedy.

In purely mechanical terms, what the alternative practitioner has done is more or less the same as the orthodox doctor. He's told him to relax, take things easy, cut down on the excesses. If the herbal preparation has any genuine pharmaceutical properties then there's no philosophical difference between offering it and the aspirin; if it has no such properties then it's at best a placebo and at worst – as we'll see later on

41

– harmful. If he's offered a massage – which might have taken the form of reflexology (i.e. a foot massage) or aromatherapy (i.e. a fragrant massage) – then it will help the patient relax sufficiently so that he will leave the surgery feeling calmer and more composed than when he went in, although it's arguable whether that tranquillity will last through the next, stressed working day. It's probable, though, that while the doctor's advice, offered after six minutes of detached consultation, was interpreted by the patient as an act of dismissal, the same advice from the concerned therapist offered after an hour of respectful consultation will be seen as an act of acceptance – acceptance of the patient's illness, discomfort, worries, insecurities. The chances are greater that the patient will change his habits as a result of that consultation and, to that extent at least, the alternative therapist has got results which the orthodox doctor hasn't.

So if that's the case, what's my objection to alternativism?

If the alternativists in that situation were honest, I'd have none at all. If they said, 'Look, we've developed some useful psychological techniques to help people get some control back over their lives, feel as if they're being taken seriously, lose – however temporarily – their sense of alienation,' then I'd have no problem, and in fact there are plenty of psychologists and psychotherapists who say precisely that, if not in so many words. I'd even accept it if they added as a rider something like 'Yes, there are some props we use, some of which have a pharmaceutical value but most of which rely on a proven placebo effect.'

The problems arise when the substantial but essentially modest claims made by the alternativists are taken a stage further – when they say that their techniques can cure organic disease. They can't. As I'll go on to demonstrate, in terms of disease most of the techniques simply don't offer anything other than a placebo, and there are plenty of illnesses, many of them serious, where a placebo isn't up to the job. As a remedy for the sort of illness that orthodox medicine would treat with drugs or surgery, for instance, homeopathy simply doesn't work. And there's no equivocation here. It's not a case of the jury being out on homeopathy, or homeopathy working only for the less worrying illnesses, or too little research on homeopathy having been carried out to determine its real potential: it doesn't work.

The same goes for a score of other remedial and diagnostic therapies. Applied kinesiology doesn't work, nor does iridology or chakra healing or cranial osteopathy or psychic surgery or crystal therapy or Kirlian photography or anthroposophical medicine or radionics or shiatsu. Of the therapies which involve ingesting substances – herbalism, naturopathy, some of the Eastern medical systems – they work only inasmuch as some of those substances have a provable pharmacological effect which involves the same chemical and biochemical principles as orthodox medicine.

(Interestingly, most alternative therapists agree with me on this. Or at least they agree that the therapies which aren't the ones they practise are useless. I showed a draft of the above to a homeopath, who was outraged that I'd listed his discipline alongside that of Kirlian photography which he described as 'patent nonsense'. A reflexologist told me that it was ridiculous to include such fringe practices as crystal therapy and anthroposophical medicine alongside her own therapy and a herbalist told me that although some of his best friends and colleagues at his therapy centre are homeopaths he has no time for that therapy's principles at all.)

But I return to the basic question: even if these therapies are worthless beyond offering the basic benefits I describe above, what harm do they do?

The harm is manifold. At a basic moral level it is, of course, wrong to tell lies. I use the word 'lie' quite purposefully because it's the word alternativists are happy to use when discussing what many of them perceive as the conspiracy of orthodox medicine. It's not a word that representatives of the orthodoxy tend to use, but then of late that orthodoxy has taken to pussyfooting around the subject. The British Medical Association, for instance, is full of doctors who believe that there is no rational basis at all to many of the therapies which their patients tell them about, but they recognise that we live in a consumerist society and that telling their patients that the crystal therapy they read about in their morning paper has no

43

basis in fact whatsoever might sound spiteful or self-serving. When the House of Lords produced its report on complementary and alternative medicine at the end of 2000, it found that most of the therapies it looked at were useless and yet it reported that fact in such painfully diplomatic language that many papers reporting on their lordships' views assumed they actually supported therapies which in fact had been dismissed as nonsense.

I'm not pretending that all, or even most, alternative therapists purposely lie to their customers, nor do I pretend that there aren't large areas of orthodox medicine in which patients are told things which are either not true or not proven. I'm pretty certain that most homeopaths really do believe that their discipline is firmly rooted in reality, that they can cure organic disease with their preparations. I'm equally certain that when I had a reflexology massage for the first time at a health spa in Florida in the late Eighties, the man working away at my feet really did believe what he told me about meridians and toxins. Equally, I'm sure there is a small but substantial number of practitioners – especially in therapies aimed at specific illnesses – who are out-and-out confidence tricksters who know that their therapies don't work but take the money anyway.

But the moral argument isn't my main problem. After all, there are numbers of industries in the business of telling lies for a living, from the outright liars of the tobacco industry, who continued to insist there was no conclusive evidence to show that their products caused cancer long after – as internal memos showed – they'd discovered just that evidence for themselves, to the fibbers and hyperbolists of the advertising and PR industries. If alternativists were just another self-serving constituency picking through the evidence to find the bits which suited their cause, exaggerating their successes and ignoring the failures, making the fallacious leaps which add two and two to give five, I'd be happy to leave them alone to get on with it.

But they go further than that. The lies of alternativism can, at worst, make people ill and, more often, stop them from getting better.

The case of Cameron Ayres is a basic example. He was born in south London in 2000 with a congenital condition which affected his metabolism and rendered him intolerant to certain foods. It was a rare illness, but an eminently treatable one using orthodox methods which, as it happens, don't involve drugs or surgery but a simple dietary routine. Unfortunately, Cameron's father treated the baby on the basis of what homeopathy told him was the cause of those particular symptoms. Cameron died shortly after being taken to the casualty department of the local hospital, screaming, with swollen testicles and an enlarged liver.

Of course, when the case made the papers, the homeopaths were lining up to explain how this really wasn't the fault of homeopathy, that another homeopathic doctor would have seen that this case was one where orthodox medicine might have been more successful, that homeopathy shouldn't be regarded as a therapy which lets babies die needlessly.

And in truth the Cameron Ayres case is a rarity – although most doctors can relate equivalent cases of such crass and blinkered stupidity. But to say that this was a case that should have been treated by orthodox methods is to make a nonsense of holistic medicine. All holistic therapies are based on the premise of each individual's uniqueness. Just as the cause of my headache isn't the cause of your headache, so the cause of my screaming baby's swollen organs isn't the cause of your screaming baby's swollen organs. Any orthodox paediatric specialist who had looked at Cameron would have known pretty quickly what the symptoms represented. The symptoms weren't a function of the baby's lifestyle or of his temperament: they were a straightforward biochemical response to a specific physiological disorder. The problem for the holistic therapies, of course, is that as soon as you start attaching particular symptoms to particular illnesses, the idea of holism goes out of the consulting-room window.

Where, on the pavement below, it will meet any number of other mindless theories.

Chapter Four

As I wrote at the start of this book, it's not my intention or even my desire to defend the medical establishment, for there is much of it which is indefensible. Parts of that establishment still have the mindset of Sir Lancelot Spratt in Richard Gordon's *Doctor in the House* novels of half a century ago: patients are little more than an encumbrance upon the doctors who treat them; knowledge is something better kept from the patients, who, let's be honest, couldn't understand it even if it were divulged to them; consultation is strictly a one-way process. There are still too many medical schools where it's considered wussy to teach the students how best to talk to anxious patients or deal with the worries behind their strictly medical problems, and there are still too many doctors who long for the days when they were regularly flown by pharmaceutical companies to Caribbean islands, there to take part in phoney conferences which had no greater medical value than persuading them to use NHS cash to prescribe Brand X rather than Brand Y.

And then, of course, there are the pharmaceutical companies themselves, which thanks to the magic of the global free market will always be prepared to spend more money researching cures for the income-generating minor illnesses which afflict the well-off rather than those for the fatal diseases which wipe out the poor.

But don't get me started. That establishment isn't what this book is about. Having said which, it's impossible to talk about the alternative-medicine establishment – and, yes, there is one – without discussing the orthodox establishment, for much of the argument in favour of alternative medicine is based on the simplistic argument which says that alternativism must be good simply because the orthodoxy can be so bad.

More, that argument talks about a medical conspiracy against patients. The case – and this is a distillation of numerous versions of it as they've been put to me over the years – goes something like this.

Orthodox medicine is big business. Throughout the developed world doctors are among the most highly paid members of society and form a professional elite which is able to control the economics of an industry which annually turns over hundreds of billions of pounds, dollars, marks and yen. But powerful as are the doctors themselves, they are in thrall to the medical research establishment, controlled on the one hand by the money-grabbing multinational pharmaceutical companies and on the other by an academic caste which allows to stand only those truths which fit its self-serving view of reality.

In order to uphold this establishment, alternativism cannot be allowed to gain any real foothold. It's against the vested interests of the pharmaceutical companies to encourage the sick to use 'traditional' remedies, or any remedies, come to that, which haven't been developed and patented by those companies: generally speaking remedies involving naturally occurring substances are unpatentable and thus incapable of being monopolised by the pharmaceutical companies to help swell their already engorged treasuries and those of their bleating and amoral shareholders.

You don't have to be a paid-up member of the Socialist Workers' Party or a twitching conspiracy theorist to accept some or even much of this first part of the argument. Yes: the drug companies are in it for the money. If AIDS, for instance, were a disease only of sub-Saharan Africa then, despite the fact that it affects and kills some millions each year, I doubt whether the big drug companies would be spending so many millions on researching a cure. They don't, after all, spend that sort of money developing treatments for malaria or bilharzia because, unlike AIDS, those diseases tend not to affect middle-class Europeans and Americans with money to spend on pharmaceutical drugs.

And, yes, academic researchers tend, for obvious reasons, to go where the research grants are. Despite the massive media coverage of, say St John's wort as 'nature's Prozac', the amount of time and money being spent in evaluating its therapeutic possibilities is rather less than was spent on developing science's Prozac or its new pharmacological relatives.

The alternativists' fantasies start when they take this economic thesis a step further. It goes like this.

The medical establishment, knowing full well the curative powers of – *insert name of miracle remedy/therapy* – conspires to keep it from the public. If they can't actually ban the treatment (and in America particularly the FDA has outlawed a number of alternative cures for, especially, cancer, to the extent where those promoting them can end up behind bars), they will try and pour sufficient academic scorn on it to keep a confused public coming back to the orthodoxy for their expensive treatments. Oncologists would prefer, says this theory, to see a million patients die of cancer than to admit that Essiac, say, or Gerson therapy works. But the orthodox establishment is even more cynical than this: not only do they know that alternative therapies work, but they also know that their own expensive and misguided therapies don't.

I am not, I promise you, exaggerating here. One US comic-book guide[*] to the medical conspiracy against curing cancer, for instance, lists the three orthodox approaches to cancer treatment, thus:

Three approved paths to the graveyard
CUT! Surgery is only a stopgap, mutilating measure that cannot remove the cause of cancer, but it may even hasten its spread!
BURN! Radiation destroys both cancer and healthy cells!

[*] Included – without provenance – in the Questionable Cancer Therapies section of *www.quackwatch.com*.

Rather, X-rays induce cancer and weaken resistance!
POISON! Drugs do not cure and have bad effects!
All of these methods are part of a multi-million dollar
death-mill!
1,000 Americans per day DIE of CANCER! 1 in 4 persons,
2 of 3 families, 53 million now living will get CANCER!

Even allowing for the comic-book grammar and the reliance
on exclamation marks, this is complete nonsense: almost
every fact in the piece is not a fact at all but, at the very best,
a half-truth. But the rant neatly, if rather hysterically, sums up
the nature of the supposed conspiracy: the medical establishment is not only withholding working remedies from us, but
it is using false and dangerous remedies of its own, which are
bound to kill cancer patients.

If there is such a conspiracy, then it's a hell of a big one.
Let's consider what its nature would be.

Let's start by taking the more paranoid conspiracists at
their word, and assume that this isn't just a matter of ignorance or misguidedness on the part of some doctors, but that
there is a real conspiracy to withhold the truth from the
public. Of course, the deal with conspiracies is that everyone
who's in on them has to be complicit in keeping the secret.
One loose mouth and the conspiracy fails.

Allow me a whimsical comparison for a moment. If you've
ever watched the early Bond films you will have been struck
by the nature of the villain's secret lair – a Caribbean island
converted into a futuristic fortress full of impossibly high-tech
weaponry, say – from which he plans to take over the world.
And if you've thought about it for more than a couple of
seconds, you'll have realised that the fiction is not so much in
the impossible nature of the weaponry but in the nature of the
fortress's secrecy. It's hard enough to build a conservatory in
London without planning permission and keeping the fact a
secret from the council: imagine building a multi-billion-
dollar fortress without word getting out. Imagine making sure
that all those hundreds of concrete pourers and plasterers and
metal fabricators and the men who rig up the dozens of

electronic doors which snap open with that phhh-ppp! sound and the ones who paint everything that forbidding shade of world-domination grey never tell a soul that the reason they've not been able to turn out for the local darts team for the past year or so is because they've been stuck on an island 3,000 miles away building a secret fortress. Now imagine recruiting all those hundreds of men and women who make the private army which gets blown to smithereens by Bond and his chums in the last scene. How do you keep them quiet? And, having kept them from selling their story to the *Sun*, how do you also make sure that they don't say a word to their gabby mum back in Liverpool or Des Moines?

It is, of course, impossible. But slightly less impossible than maintaining the secrecy that would be needed to keep the medical conspiracy against consumer health going for all these years. All you'd need is just one disenchanted doctor or nurse or radiologist to stand up and tell the world how everyone he or she works with really knows that orthodox medicine is a scam, that it can't and doesn't work, that it's merely a way of keeping GlaxoSmithKlein and Bayer in the manner to which they've become accustomed, and it would all be over. Juts one doctor who said that all those medical conferences around the world consisted of researchers and doctors slyly winking at each other and tapping the sides of their noses in the knowledge that it was all so much make-believe, just one researcher who described how there were days when she and her colleagues couldn't work for giggling at the nonsense they knew they were all perpetrating.

But as unlikely as that is, even a less outrageous conspiracist fantasy stops working when it comes up against reality.

Why, for instance, do people become doctors or nurses or join any of the auxiliary medical professions? Yes, of course some do it for the money or the power, although there are probably easier ways a bright student can find to make a moderately good living than by studying every hour God gives at a medical school, working eighty-five-hour weeks as a junior doctor and eventually, after ten or twenty years getting a cushy job treating gullible dowagers in his Harley Street consulting rooms. And while it might be that the doctors are in it for the power or money, it's unlikely that their presumed co-conspirators, working long hours for low wages as nurses or physiotherapists, would have the same motivation.

Generally speaking, people become doctors because, among other reasons, they want to heal the sick. Of course even this apparently selfless motive might not be quite as it appears, and well this side of Harold Shipman there are plenty of examples of doctors who get off on the power which their medical skills and knowledge give them. It is a cliché that doctors like to play God and, as is so often the case, clichés become clichés because they contain some truth. But it's this very truth which works against the conspiracy theory. The conspiracy theory which says the medical establishment wants to prolong the suffering of the sick assumes a doctoring class which is not only without morality, but is also without ego, without vanity, without greed.

Let's take, as an example, Essiac. Let's assume for the time being that it's all its proponents say it's cracked up to be: a simple, safe and effective cure for cancer. And not just for one cancer, or a few cancers, but for all cancers. Give Essiac to a patient with cancer and the cancer will go away. Essiac, according to its believers, is just one of the substances which the medical conspiracy is keeping away from dying cancer patients like me.

Now imagine that you're a doctor who deals with cancer patients. Your reputation is based entirely on your ability to cure your patients of their cancer. If people keep on coming to you with cancer and dying of it, you will be doing a bad job. Your self-esteem will be pretty dismal, your status among your fellow doctors will be low. Like most people, you would be happier doing your job well rather than badly. You come across Essiac. You discover that if you give it to your patients their cancer is cured.

So what do you do? Do you carry on with the cover-up, maintaining the fiction that Essiac has no curative effect on cancer? Or do you decide that, whatever your colleagues say, whatever the rules written on the back of your World Medical Conspiracy membership card, you are going to be the first cancer doctor to cure all cancers? After all, you're a doctor and in the eyes of the conspiracists that makes you venal, power-hungry, greedy, vain. What could better feed all those crazed traits than getting world fame as the discoverer of a cure for cancer? And after all – and let's remember the Bond villain and his island redoubt – you'd only need one doctor to do it; just one of the millions of doctors around the world who could announce that while his colleagues using orthodox methods were getting results 50 or 60 per cent of the time, he – Dr Wonderful – was curing 80, 90 or 100 per cent of the grateful wretches coming to him with their tumours.

And if one doctor was getting better than average results from using Essiac (or any of the dozens of other alternative therapies listed under the Questionable Cancer Therapies section on *www.quackwatch.com*) how long would it be before another doctor joined in, and another and another?

Ah yes, say the alternativists: but that isn't the way the orthodoxy works. Even if the truth is made obvious to them, the medical establishment will refuse point-blank to see it. Look, they say, at the case of the peptic ulcer and the bacterium *helicobacter pylori*. *H. pylori* is one of the alternativists' favourite case-studies and the one most regularly brought out and dusted off to demonstrate orthodox medicine's resistance to change and the drug companies' complicity in that resistance.

For most of the twentieth century it was a medical given that peptic ulcers were caused by such things as stress, spicy foods and riotous living. For much of that century the treatment prescribed for ulcers was so standard as to have become part of the language of the sit-com, with the harassed executive drinking a glass of milk to relieve the pain of his ulcer, which was caused by whatever comic situation we were being treated to. Ulcers were not only common, but were common among well-off Westerners, and it could only be a matter of time before the drug companies came up with an expensive treatment for them. The treatment, which appeared in the mid-Seventies, was ranitidine, which didn't cure the ulcer but which prevented histamine from stimulating gastric activity.

And then in 1982 a couple of Australian researchers, Drs J. Robin Warren and Barry Marshall, discovered the connection between peptic ulcers and the bacterium and it's now understood that neither spicy food nor stress causes ulcers and that between 70 and 80 per cent of peptic ulcers are caused by H. pylori. Which would be just another tale of medical discovery were it not – as the alternativists are so keen to point out – for the length of time it took to convince the medical establishment of the connection.

I have some dozens of medical books around my office: look up any of them published before the mid-Nineties and you'll find peptic ulcers described the old-fashioned way, as a disorder brought on by too many prawn vindaloos or too many late-night meetings. The treatment, these books go on to say, is with ranitidine. The alternativists are right: it did take the medical establishment an awfully long time to accept the H. pylori connection and, ten years after the original research, gastro-intestinal specialists were still prescribing the old, expensive drugs, performing the operations based on the presumed incurability of certain varieties of ulcer and so on. Why did it take them so long to come around to the new way of thinking? Because, yes, vested interests were involved. And not just those of the drug company which had invested so much in developing ranitidine and which would have had only a decade to recoup their investment had the industry listened to Warren and Marshall from the off: doctors, often almost as vain and self-serving as the alternativists make them out to be, not only hated to admit that they'd been wrong for all these years, but hated the need to replace the old, esoteric science of the peptic ulcer with a new, simple science which said this was something any GP could prescribe an antibiotic for.

It wasn't until 1994 – a full twelve years after the original research appeared – that the US ulcer industry convened a consensus-development conference on H. pylori at which they agreed that, yes, this was the cause of most peptic ulcers and that, yes, they shouldn't have been so rude about Warren and Marshall, upon whose heads vast amounts of self-serving scorn had been poured in the intervening years.

All of which looks, at first glance, just the sort of thing which demonstrates the rightness of the conspiracists' case. In fact it demonstrates, if anything at all, more or less the opposite – and not least because, ironically enough, it demonstrates a 'science'-based therapy involving bugs and pills replacing a 'lifestyle'-based therapy which, in its reliance on nutrition, lack of stress and good living habits, could almost come straight from any alternativist's book of healthy living. The old guard *did* come round to the new way of thinking and although twelve years is a long time if you've got an ulcer gnawing away at your guts, it's a relatively short time in terms of medical research. Moreover, it changed its mind without any apparent reference to the companies which were making good money from the recently patented ulcer drugs – drugs which earn their patent-holders rather less money in their new incarnation as prophylaxis against gastritis which may be caused by certain painkillers used in the treatment of other-illnesses.

The fact is that, although the alternativists like to portray the orthodoxy as hidebound and scared of change, much of the evidence suggests that the opposite is true. Look through any edition of one of the hundreds of medical journals produced around the world and you'll notice two things. The first is medicine's fondness for novelty: the cancer hospital I attend has some dozens of new and unproven techniques under trial – including a few based on substances which would be familiar to herbalists. The second is the willingness of ortho-dox researchers to trash each other's research and methods. I've just picked up a copy of the *British Medical Journal* at random and found that of the eight papers published in it, two reveal that particular orthodox treatments are useless.

Compare this with almost any 'traditional' alternative medical therapy. The alternativists complain – against the evidence – about the orthodoxy's hidebound unwillingness to change, while at the same time taking a perverse pride in the antiquity of their own techniques. I've never come across a herbalist who has revealed that a remedy used by his profes-sional forebears has been discovered, after all, not to work, or a homeopath complaining that his craft is still stuck in the rut ploughed by homeopathy's founder two hundred years ago.

Nor, come to that, have I ever heard an alternativist admit that the vested interests of the heterodoxy are just as great as those of the orthodoxy. And they're as great for much the same reasons: money and pride.

Alternative medicine is big business. True, it's not nearly as big as orthodox medicine, but it's certainly progressed beyond the level where we could think of it as a ragbag collection of gentle and slightly impoverished practitioners working from their back rooms for peanuts. It's difficult to gauge just how much the business is worth in Britain because there's no agreed definition of which parts of the patent-medicine business count as 'alternative'. There are plenty of alternativists, for instance, who tout vitamins as part of a curative regime, but most assessments of the value of the industry wouldn't include the millions spent on vitamin supplements at high street chemists. But generally speaking a conservative estimate of the amount spent on Complementary and Alternative Medicine (CAM) in Britain in 2000 is about £1.6 billion,[*] with about 50,000 Britons styling themselves as CAM practitioners and 10,000 statutory registered health professionals offering CAM as well as their orthodox therapies.[**] In America the industry is bigger still, running at about $27 billion according to evidence given to the House of Lords Select Committee on Science and Technology.

And just as the orthodox industry has its two poles, with the kindly, overworked GP at one end and the profit-crazed drug company at the other, so the modern alternative business is fuelled by the same need to move product as any other industry. Just as the local GP might disapprove of the actions of the companies whose drugs he prescribes, so the local homeopaths might disdain the mass-produced do-it-yourself

---

[*] E. Ernst and A. White, 'The BBC Survey of Complementary Medicine Use in the UK', *Complementary Therapies in Medicine*, 8 (March 2000), pp. 32–6.

[**] S. Mills and W. Peacock, *Professional Organisation of Complementary and Alternative Medicine in the UK, 1997: A Report to the Department of Health* (University of Exeter, 1997).

homeopathic remedies filling the shelves of the local branch of Boots, where they're sold by a druggist whose own pharmacological training often makes him an unwilling champion of the alternative method.

But that doesn't change the nature of the vested interest. (And somebody even more cynical than I am might add that an overworked GP might be glad that Boots sells homeopathic remedies and keeps a few people with minor chronic complaints out of his surgery, while a homeopath who gets paid only by the consultation would be out of pocket whenever a potential patient goes the DIY route.)

But even if there was some good economic reason why the financial imperatives which apply to the medical orthodoxy don't for some reason apply equivalently to the alternative industry, the real vested interest is in the practitioners themselves.

Over the past few years whenever I've written in the press about alternativism I've had e-mails and letters from aggrieved practitioners who think I'm treating them unfairly. Occasionally I used to get into friendly correspondences with them and we would spend a while swapping facts and prejudices. But I've stopped. The exchanges may be enjoyable, but they're pointless. I don't pretend for a moment that my rhetorical powers are any better than those of the average homeopath or naturopath, but there comes a point in the exchange when I've delivered what I regard as proofs of the inadequacy of their therapies but when the response is simply denial. The denial usually takes the form of a sentence like 'There's no point in offering you proof of how homeopathy works: you simply wouldn't believe it because you've closed your mind to the possibility,' and it only occurred to me relatively recently that I was asking the impossible of my adversaries – in, it has to be admitted, exactly the same way as they are asking the impossible of the orthodoxy.

My last correspondent, for instance, was a homeopath in the north of Britain. He'd trained some years ago at one of the grander homeopathic colleges and had spent years building up his practice, sitting on committees which aimed to regulate the practice of his craft, participating in research trials, generally becoming part of the homeopathic establishment. If I believed in homeopathy I couldn't imagine a better way of leading one's professional life. But in asking him to consider the arguments against homeopathy I was asking him to consider that which he couldn't possible consider. I was asking him to say to himself – and to his colleagues, patients and the community at large – 'Everything I've devoted my professional life to for the past eighteen years was based on a series of false premises and fallacies. All the work I've put into refining my skills, building up my practice, spreading the good word about homeopathy, has been wasted. I have a head full of knowledge about a subject where all knowledge is invalid. I have wasted my time.'

And how many of us, orthodox or heterodox, would be willing to say that to ourselves? What are the chances of the College of Homeopathy meeting together one day and passing a resolution saying 'It's all so much nonsense' and disbanding itself?

No more, you may say, than there is any chance of the Royal College of General Practitioners passing the equivalent motion, which would be fair comment were it not for the fact that even if the orthodoxy doesn't pass the resolution which will wipe it out, it is willing – when pushed, screaming – to meet in convocation and agree, for instance, that it was wrong all along about peptic ulcers, or balloon angioplasty or any of the other changes in direction and belief the medical establishment has taken over the years.

Alternativists rarely make those sort of admissions.

CHAPTER FIVE

MOST OF THE time, under most circumstances, most of us are pretty clear about what is a fact and what isn't. If I point to a table and say, 'Here is a chair,' you will know that I'm probably lying: your long experience of tables and chairs and what constitutes essential tableness or chairity tells you so. Of course my describing a table as a chair may not be a matter of simple lie-telling on my part: I may be mad, or deluded, or a nominal aphasic, or I may come from some part of the country, unknown to you, where the dialect word for what you call a table is 'chair'. It may be that, although I recognise that the object was created with tableness in mind, I want to make the deeper point that because it's capable of being sat on its function is ambivalent.

But even if I allow the example to spin off into such metaphysical realms here on the page, both you and I know that there's a general consensus about what a table is and what a chair is, and the chances are that we can come to some agreement about what the object is and what we should call it. For all that semioticists and deconstructuralists and post-modernists tell us about the fickle nature of meaning, at the most fundamental and everyday level we know that a shop which opens for business with 'We Sell Only Chairs' emblazoned over its door will go broke pretty soon if all it stocks is tables.

But what if, having established that we agree on what a chair is, I take you into a furniture warehouse, show you a massive room filled to the rafters with chairs, and tell you there are precisely 10,000 chairs stacked there? And what if I go on to say that you can have the chairs for a knock-down £10 each and that as soon as you write me a cheque for £100,000 they're all yours. (No, I don't know why you'd want 10,000 chairs. A particularly flash bar mitzvah, a new branch of IKEA, a large bonfire: this analogy still has some way to run, so use your imagination and bear with me, will you?)

You start to count them.

'No,' I say, 'you really should take my word for it. That's what ten thousand chairs looks like.'

Well, yes, it may be what 10,000 chairs looks like, but you've never seen that number of chairs before, and while you could judge the truth of 'There are ten chairs,' or even, possibly, 'There are a hundred chairs' with a quick glance around the room, and know that in those circumstances you may be only a chair or two out, at this level you really have no idea whether you're looking at 5,000 chairs or 15,000 chairs. You simply don't have the experience of chair-number-assessing to take the risk of signing that cheque.

So how do you ascertain how many chairs there are? You could, I suppose, use your experience, not of chair-assessing, but of people-assessing. What are the chances of a chair-seller lying to you? Have you been lied to by chair-sellers in the past? Have you been lied to by *this* chair-seller in the past? Is your view of chair-sellers skewed by the fact that your mother ran off with the manager of the local branch of Chairs 'R' Us when you were a child? Or, come to that, by a beloved uncle being president of the local chapter of the British Chair Fanciers Association?

Obviously the only answer is to count the chairs. It is the most logical, the most accurate way of determining their number. Who can argue with that?

Well, it seems the chair-seller can. I understand, I say, that counting works pretty well in many circumstances, but it's a myth put about by self-serving mathematicians that it's the *only* way of assessing a number. Only the other week, I say, I had 2,000 chairs to get rid of and I made the mistake of allowing the customer to count them. And what do you know? The customer counted 1,700!

So that must mean, you say, that there were only 1,700 chairs.

'No,' I say. 'There were absolutely two thousand of them.' Reasonably enough, you ask how I could possibly know that without counting them.

'Because,' I say, 'I am a seller of chairs. I know these things. What's more, I brought half a dozen fellow chair-sellers along to give a look over the chairs, and they all agreed there were two thousand of them. Between us, our experience, our instinct, our feeling for chairs and numbers must be worth more than mere counting.'

Eventually, though, you persuade me that the only way you're going to take all these chairs off my hands is if I let you count them. You start: 'One, two, three . . .' And I start too. 'Fifty-six!' I shout. 'Four hundred and seventy-three. Nine. Three thousand two hundred and twelve . . .' You complain that it's impossible to count the chairs properly while I'm shouting numbers at random. I stop. You start again: 'One, two, three . . .' I turn on a tape deck from which a voice gently murmurs, 'Ten thousand chairs. There are ten thousand chairs. You will count ten thousand chairs . . .'

Eventually you stop. 'Look,' you say. 'I'm prepared to buy your chairs. I want to buy your chairs. But I'll only buy them if you'll let me count them and, what's more, let me count them without distraction. OK?'

And I say, 'Well if you're going to be unreasonable about it, you can go and buy your chairs somewhere else.'

Which isn't that far removed from the attitude most alternativists have towards assessing the validity of their therapies.

The obvious way of discovering whether homeopathy or herbalism (or, of course, antibiotics or cough medicine) works is simply, as it were, to count the chairs – to give the treatment to a number of suitable patients and see what happens to them. Take a hundred people with high blood pressure, give them all Black Haw – one of the traditional herbal remedies for high blood pressure – and measure their blood pressure again. If the blood pressure falls then you can say that there's some good chance that Black Haw lowers blood pressure. Easy.

Well, no. Not quite so easy. Hypertension – high blood pressure – can be caused by any number of diseases and by none at all. It can be a symptom of a clogged arterial system or of an impending exam, a dodgy kidney or a failed love affair. Thus far alternativists would agree with the orthodoxy: at this level, at least, we are all individuals and our symptoms are those of our individual physiological situations. And while an alternativist might tell you that treating the symptoms caused by 'blood pressure of the menopause' would suggest the use of Black Cohosh while 'high blood pressure where there is nerve excitability' calls for valerian, a medical doctor would be more likely to differentiate between essential hypertension – i.e. hypertension where there is no apparent cause, as is the case 90 per cent of the time – and hypertension which results from some organic disorder or another, and either treat that disorder itself or prescribe one or other of the drugs which lowers blood pressure.

Either way, you can't simply test for the efficacy of the drug, or the herb, by picking hypertensive subjects at random. You have, as it were, to make sure that all your chairs are chairs before you start counting them. What's more, you have to make sure that nobody is standing by your shoulder shouting random numbers as you do the counting, or doing anything else which will influence the number you finish up with.

Provided that you do not believe, like me in my chair-selling guise, that there is some alternative way of assessing the number of chairs other than counting them, then the best accepted way of testing for the efficacy of medical therapies – orthodox or alternative – is the randomised double-blind trial.

There is nothing particularly esoteric about the reasoning behind such trials, although some alternativists will tell you either that the method is unnecessarily complicated, or that it carries its own bias, or that it is inappropriate in many of the cases where alternative therapies work best. Some alternativists whose therapies proudly dispense with any scientific basis at all will tell you that such trials are meaningless because they have no spiritual dimension.

Meanwhile, in the rational world, the randomised double-blind trial is an attempt to get somewhere near an objective assessment of the facts without being influenced by the prejudices of the researcher, the subject or any of the other hundred and one elements which can influence the outcome of such a trial.

Let's take as an example the use of arnica.

Arnica is a fairly common, undistinguished yellow plant of the aster family; it grows wild, is mildly toxic in large quantities and occasionally turns up in suburban garden rockeries looking sulphurous and droopy. It's also one of the plants most commonly used by herbalists and homeopaths for anything from mild bruising to muscle strain to post-operative pain relief to 'shock following bereavement'. It was first used, depending on who you believe, by Swiss mountaineers who needed to relieve their fatigued muscles, or by the twelfth-century abbess of Mount St Rupert, St Hildegard of Bingen, who wrote three works on the Book of Revelations. A herbalist and a homeopath will use the plant in different ways (not least because the herbalist's treatment will actually contain some of the arnica while the homeopath's will contain only the 'memory' of the arnica), but in principle they're agreed that it works well with aches, sprains and bruising.

Arnica is also one of the 'natural' treatments which have crossed the consumer barrier from alternative to, well, if not orthodox then mainstream. Most high-street pharmacies carry at least a couple of arnica creams and I know a number of mothers of young children who while forswearing alternative medicine in almost every other circumstance regularly use arnica creams on their children's playground scrapes. They've always struck me as the equivalent of those people who say, 'Of course astrology is a lot of mumbo-jumbo, but you have to admit that Patric Walker was strangely gifted.'

So how do you test the proposition that a homeopathic preparation of arnica does the trick?

The easy answer is to give a preparation of arnica to a large number of people with bruises, bumps and strains and see what they think of its effects. Sure, that would be an entirely subjective assessment, but then with such minor wounds subjectivity is usually good enough: deciding whether something hurts enough to take the day off work or skip school is often a pretty subjective matter. But still it doesn't tell us anything more about arnica than that some people think it works for them. To get a proper assessment you need to start off with a group of people with similar ailments (it's difficult to make any objective assessment when you're comparing, say, toothache to a sprained wrist) and divide them into two halves. You give one half the arnica and another a placebo, which is to say a preparation which looks identical to the arnica but has no active ingredient whatsoever.

But even then you don't have a fully objective test. How do you divide the group into two? You certainly can't ask the participants which group they'd prefer to go into: that way there's a chance that those who believe in the healing power of arnica will choose the arnica group, while those who believe in the healing power of placebos . . . you see the problem. Nor can you ask the researchers to make the division: there's no guarantee that however objective a researcher believes him or herself to be, they won't skew the results by, say, subconsciously choosing those who somehow look unsympathetic to alternative medicine for one group or the other. Hence randomisation.

The idea isn't a new one: it was first suggested in the mid-seventeenth century by a Dutch physician, John Baptista van Helmont.[*] In those days the standard cure for fevers (under which broad heading you could include most bacterial and viral diseases) was bloodletting, in which either the skin would be cut with a knife and allowed to bleed or leeches would be allowed to suck blood from the patient. It was a nasty and painful treatment, with insult being added to injury by the fact that it didn't really work. Indeed, it says something about the blind faith of the average orthodox doctor – and this was, after all, orthodox procedure right into the nineteenth century – that they carried on doing it regardless of the fact that they must have seen it wasn't any use. (In fact, it was because of the gore, pain and

---

[*] J.B. van Helmont, *Oriatrike or, Physick Refined* (London: Lodowick Loyd, 1662), p. 526.

inefficacy of bloodletting that Dr Samuel Hahnemann devised homeopathy not so very long after van Helmont was working.)

Van Helmont issued a wager to his fellow doctors. He bet them three hundred florins that if he took one group of fever-sufferers and treated them without bloodletting and they took an equivalent group and gave them the standard treatment, fewer of his patients would die. Importantly, in terms of medical history, he suggested that the patients should be chosen 'by lot', which is to say randomly. There is no record of whether the bet was ever taken up or, if it was, who won it, but certainly the principle was established – even if it wasn't acted on for some hundreds of years.

These days the randomisation is usually carried out by computer and because of the double-blind nature of the trial, only the computer knows who has been chosen to take what.

Van Helmont's test would have been randomised, but it wouldn't have been blind. A single-blind test means that the researcher knows into which group each subject has been put, but this, too, can cause bias, hence the value placed on double-blind trials in which neither the researcher nor the subject knows whether the drug they're taking is the real thing or the placebo.

Again, this is the only way to stop unconscious bias. In one trial[*] to test the efficacy of Therapeutic Touch or TT (a healing therapy used mainly in the United States) researchers attempted to gauge the claim that therapists can emit a Human Energy Field or HEF. The researchers wanted to see whether subjects could guess with a better accuracy than chance would dictate whether TT practitioners' hands were near their own and thus emitting this HEF. They went to some lengths to cover the hands and to shield researchers from the subjects, so that only when the subject heard the researcher say 'ready' would they say whether they thought the HEF-emitting hand was near theirs.

---

[*] R. Long, P. Bernhardt and W. Evans, 'Perception of Conventional Sensory Cures as an Alternative to the Postulated "Human Energy Field" of Therapeutic Touch', *Science Meets Alternative Medicine*, (New York: Prometheus Books, 2000), p. 165.

Except that it turned out that even with these safeguards in place the subjects subconsciously picked up cues which were equally subconsciously given by the researchers. Researchers would unconsciously look in the direction of a hand which was placed over the subject's hand, or lean in a particular way on the table while they were covering the hand.

The reason such apparently tiny influences are important is because very often the results themselves are a matter of tiny differences between outcomes. One of the reasons there is still so much argument about the efficacy of homeopathy, for instance, is because some of the trials which its proponents say show the therapy works actually show a very small variation from what one would expect if the therapy didn't work. As we'll see later on, very often the results of scientific – or purportedly scientific – trials of alternative remedies can be divided into three groups: those which show the remedy to work, those which show the remedy not to work, and those where the trial was not sufficiently well designed to make the call.

Thus in one overview of eight different trials of homeo-pathically used arnica,* four of the trials showed no difference at all between using arnica and using a placebo. Of the other four, each of them seemed to show some small but significant benefits for the patients using the arnica treatment but, as Professor Ernst notes in his summary, 'Most of these studies were burdened with severe methodological flaws.'

Most of the homeopaths I've spoken to tend to describe these objections in terms of moving the goalposts. Their protestation goes like this: scientists are forever demanding that we submit our claims to what they insist are the only acceptable tests of whether any remedy works; we do this and show that, yes, the remedy does work. Then they say that if it shows the remedy works the test couldn't have been properly constructed. We can't win.

Which isn't how it is at all. Scientific testing – and this

---

* E. Ernst, 'Efficacy of Homeopathic Arnica – a Systematic Review of Placebo-Controlled Clinical Trials', *Journal American Medical Association*, *Arch. Surg.*, 133 (1998), pp. 1187–90.

applies whether you're testing alternative remedies or orthodox ones – means finding a way of ascertaining the truth. That involves, among other things, comparing like with like, using sufficiently large numbers of examples so that the results are meaningful, and weeding out all those factors which might influence the results.

So there we have your blue-chip standard for scientific testing: the double-blind, randomised trial. (Actually, the blue-chip standard adds the qualifier 'peer-reviewed'; a double-blind randomised trial carried out by me and my mum would have less chance of convincing the medical profession than one carried out by people who, their peers agree, know what they're doing.)

With the arnica review, for instance, one trial published in the *British Homeopathic Journal*, came out in favour of arnica as a treatment for bruising on the basis of just ten subjects being tested and gave no statistics at all.

At the other end of the scale is a trial which treated 118 patients after their wisdom teeth were extracted. All the criteria were fulfilled. The 118 patients had much the same wounds to deal with; there were objective (wound-healing, oedema, bleeding) as well as subjective (pain) determinants of how well the treatment was working, the trial was randomised and double-blind. I hardly need to say that in that trial arnica did no better than the placebo and rather worse than a standard anti-bacterial treatment given to a third group of patients.

So what objection do alternativists have to the double-blind random trial? And how can such an objection make any more sense than the chair-seller objecting that counting his chairs isn't the correct way to assess their number?

There are, of course, some trials which can never be truly random or truly blind. Last year, for instance, I was treated with chemotherapy for my cancer. At the time, the hospital was conducting a trial to see whether the therapy was more effective and better tolerated when administered in the usual three-weekly doses or in smaller amounts delivered continuously via a Hickman line into the chest. Certainly the trial was randomised: once I'd agreed to take part in it I was allotted my place as a Hickman line recipient by luck of the computerised draw. But it could hardly be either single or double blind: even if I hadn't noticed a yard of plastic tubing sticking out of my chest, my oncologist almost certainly would have. And in any case there is a difference between assessing the treatment of cancer and that of pain or bruising, for while, as I pointed out earlier, pain is a matter of subjective measurement, the size of a tumour can be measured with the oncological equivalent of a tape measure, and my knowing which half of the trial I was in would have made no difference to the result.

The alternativist argument against this sort of trial varies, depending on which alternative therapist you're talking to. Any sort of holistic practitioner might say that all trials of this type depend on the myth that you can group together large numbers of people with 'the same' illness, when in fact holism says that all illnesses are functions of the whole person, not of a particular disease or illness or trauma. Treating all wisdom-teeth patients with arnica, they say, is a ridiculous exercise because a patient is more than an inanimate object which happens to have had a tooth removed: an Arsen. Alb. type ('thin, stylish, well groomed and aristocratic looking' says one popular homeopathic text,* whose weak areas of the body include the stomach, liver, skin and heart) needs a different treatment from an Argentum nit. type ('tend to have sunken features and develop early lines and wrinkles which make them look prematurely old and mentally overtaxed'. Their weak areas include 'The left side of the body', poor things.) Thus the 'arnica type' is 'restless, hopeless and morose [and has] a morbid imagination', which suggests that using arnica to treat the missing teeth of Krusty the Klown would be a waste of time.

But valid as this argument may be (and its validity depends, of course, on the validity of the typifications), there are many arguments against the double-blind trial which have not even this dubious logic on which to rest.

---

* Drs A. Lockie and N. Geddes, *Natural Health Complete Guide to Homeopathy* (Dorling Kindersley, 2000).

One of my favourite double-blind, randomised trial stories[*] is told by Ray Hyman, Professor Emeritus of Psychology at the University of Oregon and a leading light in the US Committee for the Scientific Investigation of Claims of the Paranormal, or CSICOP. He was taking part in a double-blind test of a technique called applied kinesiology. The theory behind the technique suggests that certain substances interfere with the body's electro-chemical system and that a subject tainted by such a substance will be less able to hold his arm locked at right angles to his body than an untainted subject. It was the method used by my clinical ecologist to test my response to any number of potential allergies that afternoon in Bayswater all those years ago and is used as a cheap and cheerful diagnostic tool by all sorts of alternativists.

The test Hyman was involved in was of the body's ability to differentiate between glucose (a 'bad' sugar) and fructose (a 'good' sugar). Subjects would lie down, put a drop of glucose on their tongue and hold their arm out at right angles to their chest. The alternativists – chiropractors, in this case – would try to push the arm down to the horizontal and in almost every case they succeeded: the 'bad' sugar had apparently affected the subjects' ability to lock their arm. Then they gave the subjects fructose and tried again; this time the arms stayed locked: the 'good' sugars hadn't affected the muscles' electro-chemical systems.

The group broke for lunch and afterwards tried the experiment again, this time with the double-blind element added. A large number of test tubes were brought in, each containing either glucose or the identical-looking fructose. Each tube was labelled with a code rather than the name of the substance: only after the test would anyone – testers, testees, observers – know whether a tube contained fructose or glucose. The subjects took a drop of the liquid on their tongue and as before sometimes they were able to resist, sometimes they weren't.

The code was broken. It turned out, of course, that under the more rigorous conditions there was absolutely no connection

---

[*] *The Mischief-Making of Ideomotor Action: Science Meets Alternative Medicine* (New York: Prometheus Books, 2000), p. 110.

between the type of sugar the subjects had eaten and their ability to resist.

Hyman wrote:

> When these results were announced, the head chiropractor turned to me and said, 'You see, that is why we never do double-blind testing any more. It never works!' At first I thought he was joking. It turned out he was quite serious. Since he 'knew' that applied kinesiology works, and the best scientific method shows that it does not, then – in his mind – there must be something wrong with the scientific method.

Which is the equivalent of my claim that because I 'know' there are 2,000 chairs then if counting the chairs shows there are only 1,700 it must follow that counting is the wrong method to use to determine how many chairs there are.

On this basis I make no apology at all for using the double-blind randomised trial as the best determinant of what is true and what isn't.

You may believe that the random double-blind method is essentially faulty, and if you do then that is absolutely your prerogative. But I've yet to come across a better method of sorting out what works from what doesn't.

CHAPTER SIX

Is THERE AN alternative, then, to the sort of rigorous and standardised proof that the picky scientist demands? The only reasonable one, and the one most often offered by the alternativists, is anecdotal evidence, and indeed you'll often hear practitioners say something like, 'I don't care if it works in the lab or not: I've seen it work every day in my consulting room, and that's good enough for me.' Which, in an ideal world, would be good enough for everyone.

The problem with the sort of anecdote which goes against science, logic, rationalism or, more importantly, experimental trial – which is to say the anecdotage which scientific proof somehow can't bring itself to support – is that all too often it falls to pieces as soon as you inspect it too closely.

An example.

Not so long ago I got an e-mail from the close friend of a fifty-year-old woman with lung cancer. The doctors, she said, had given her friend 'a year to live' and on that basis she'd 'been sent home from hospital to die'. Luckily someone had told her friend about the Gerson diet. She'd tried it and her doctors just couldn't believe the results: her latest scan showed the tumours had shrunk beyond any expectation and now they wanted to write about her experiences in a professional journal.

Which at first sight seems some sort of evidence, at least, for the Gerson diet working. Without it she was going to die; using it, the chances seemed to be that she would live. Even if this wasn't a miracle cure then obviously it was having some sort of effect, wasn't it? Why should evidence like this – offered in good faith by somebody who has only the good health of her friend in mind – not to be taken just as seriously as a laboratory trial conducted by a know-it-all scientist with God only knows what axes to grind?

Here's why.

I e-mailed the friend back with just one question: if the patient was beyond the hospital's help, why were they still giving her scans? CT (computerised tomography) scans are expensive, use the skills of a number of highly trained staff and, generally speaking, are given only to those patients who are receiving some treatment at the hospital in order to determine how well that treatment is progressing.

It suggested that they were giving her friend orthodox treatment at the same time as she was taking the Gerson treatment.

The friend e-mailed back. Well, yes: as it happened they were. She was still going into the hospital each week and being given substantial doses of radiotherapy. But that was beside the point: the reason she hadn't mentioned it in the original letter was that she was sure that it was the Gerson therapy that was making the difference.

And from where the friend was watching – and the patient herself, perhaps – this made reasonable sense. Perhaps it *was* the Gerson diet.

As it happens, we have pretty good figures on the success rates for the treatment of cancer by radiotherapy. Yes, some of those on the more paranoid fringes of the Your-Evil-Doctor-Wants-You-to-Die anti-medical movement will tell you that radiotherapy has no beneficial effect whatsoever, but generally speaking we have reasonably good evidence that radiotherapy can shrink tumours, sometimes to the point of disappearance. I'm no trained radiologist, but even I could see the difference between the X-rays of my lung before and after radiotherapy, and although the tumour has since returned there's no real doubt that a single, long session on the radiotherapy table shrank the tumour in my lung to the point of invisibility. We can have, if you like, the argument about whether this is a wise or safe treatment in the long term, but there's no doubt that if my correspondent's lung was treated in the same way then there's every probability that a scan would have shown just what it did show: a diminution in the amount of cancer.

We also know that since Gerson therapy was first subject to scrutiny by the New York Board of Health in 1949, every proper investigation of its efficacy has shown that it has none whatsoever.

As for the 'year to live' business, well, I know that one pretty well too. As it happens, sensible doctors rarely give such precise figures for survival – except, of course, in television soap operas where an actor's contract has to be taken into account when making a prognosis: 'I'm terribly sorry, Mrs Tremorly, but I'm afraid your husband has a . . . bad agent. He's only got three episodes to live.' In the real world doctors know that rampant cancers sometimes slow down and slow-growing cancers sometimes get aggressive. Sometimes treatments kick in later than expected, sometimes normally successful treatments don't work at all. One of the great myths of orthodox medicine – as circulated by almost anyone who isn't a doctor, at least – is that as sciences go it's too precise for its own good, that doctors think they know everything. In fact, as most reasonably honest doctors will tell you, medicine is the most imprecise science of all and only the most reckless doctor would say something as precise as 'She has only a year to live.'

But patients, and their loved ones, have problems dealing with such equivocation. When you're lying in a hospital bed all odds are 50:50 – it may happen and then again it may not. I've been in precisely that position myself. When it turned out that surgery and radiotherapy had failed to see off my own cancer, I was offered chemotherapy. How long, I asked, would I last without the chemo? The oncologist shrugged. Who could say? Three months? Six? A year? And how long would I have if I did have the chemo? He shrugged again: there was only a small chance of the chemotherapy having any effect at all, and if it did then I was unlikely to have more than three months' remission.

For a while I translated this in my head and in my retelling as 'The doctors have given me three months to live.' They'd done no such thing, of course, but it's difficult to pass on the equivocations of doctors to friends and relatives who want absolute facts.

Yet here I am eighteen months later. The doctors are overjoyed with my progress. My friends say I must be some sort of walking medical miracle. Well, of course the doctors are overjoyed: they work in a branch of their profession where most of the time bad things happen and when once in a while a good thing happens it's hardly surprising that they want to share their professional glee with its subject. And the reason my friends think some miracle has been worked on me is because of all the time I spent telling them I had mere months to live. In fact all I am is a point on a long line of statistical points. I'd have to stay alive for a decade or two longer before I passed into the realms of even the semi-miraculous.

So let's apply all this to my correspondent's story.

Her friend has had cancer for some time. She's had an amount of treatment – surgical, chemotherapeutic, radiotherapeutic – but every time the cancer comes back. The doctors aren't hopeful, but they've decided to give her some more radiotherapy. The friend, depressed after months or years of nasty, toxic and painful treatments, expects the worst. Indeed, she's been told that if the radiotherapy doesn't work it's possible that she might not see out the year.

In a desperate attempt to find a cure where the orthodoxy can obviously find none, she tries Gerson therapy. The theory behind it, as it's explained to her, sounds a bit complicated but it seems to make some sort of sense. It talks of 'toxins' in much the same way as she's read the word used each day in her paper's 'Body and Health' section: why should it not be that the cancer is caused by those very same toxins? She takes the treatment: she drinks the daily gallon of raw fruit and vegetable juice, has the coffee enemas, embarks on the low-sodium diet. Why not? She knows, because we all seem to these days, that raw juices are 'naturally' good for us, that too much sodium is bad, that celebrities with access to the most expensive medical advice famously have enemas for all sorts of interesting reasons, some of which we can only speculate on. She may even go the whole hog and have liver extract injections and some of the other, more esoteric treatments which the late Dr Gerson and, nowadays, his daughter recommend.

And look! Just six months later and the tumour has shrunk! The doctors, who said – as the friend understood it – the patient should by rights be dead, can't believe their eyes! And given that the orthodox medicine didn't work in the past, why should the patient, or her friend, believe that it's the orthodox medicine which has worked this time?

Except that's not the true story. The story is an everyday one in oncological terms: patient has tumour, various methods are used to try to get rid of it, eventually one method – radiotherapy in this case – does the trick. Or does it for a while, at least. I haven't been back in touch with the friend because we agreed to differ about this: as far as she was concerned my asking these awkward questions showed no more than my bad grace in refusing to accept what was obviously a story of something very special and unusual. It may well be that the patient has lived well beyond the extent of the remission which she'd had when the friend got in contact with me: these things happen and the fact that I'm writing this book is some sort of demonstration of that. If I finish the book that will be a greater demonstration still, of course.

It may, on the other hand, be that, as with me, the radiation treatment had an effect for six or nine months before the tumour came back. Either way, I wouldn't be surprised if the Gerson people aren't claiming another success. However, one independent follow-up undertaken (by a naturopath, as it happens) in the 1980s showed that nineteen out of twenty traced patients had died of their cancer; the twentieth was cancerous again.

I've heard scores of anecdotes like this and have spoken to cancer specialists and writers, like Rob Buckman, who have heard hundreds. Invariably, they involve the claim that a 'miracle' alternative treatment did the trick where orthodox remedies failed.

Equally invariably it turns out that the patient was undergoing orthodox therapy at the same time or had just finished undergoing it when the alternative treatment started. And just as invariably as that it's the case that the claim for the miracle is made well within the period when the patient could normally expect remission as a result of the orthodox cure.

There are variations on the theme too. One breast-cancer sufferer wrote to me about her experience of one of the Tijuana clinics, where she'd gone after her chemotherapy in London had left her feeling wretched. After six weeks on the alternative Mexican regime she felt wonderful and the tumour had gone.

Again, anyone listening to that story with an open mind and some modicum of good grace might well hear a moving story of alternative success. Until, that is, you think about the nature of chemotherapy. It's highly toxic and makes you feel lousy. Even after the last course of the drugs it takes a few weeks for you to stop feeling lousy and often its benefits aren't apparent until some weeks after the course has finished. Using precisely the same logic I could tell you that nasty chemotherapy had no effect on my own cancer, but that six weeks after it was over and thanks to my sticking to a dietary regime of Nestlé's Build-Up, Stolichnaya and the occasional Havana cigar, I felt a hundred times better than I had under the chemo, and that while at the end of the chemotherapy I still seemed to have some tumour, by the end of the period of Build-Up, vodka and smoking I was cured. I know, I know: that's ridiculous and obviously booze and tobacco are not cancer cures. But I used precisely the same *post hoc* argument that my correspondent had used: I had a tumour; I took chemotherapy; I felt lousy; I finished the chemotherapy and I felt better and saw my tumour shrink.

If you're still a doubter, let me give you a single fact to consider. It is, I suppose I should acknowledge, an anecdote and thus by my own judgement no absolute proof, but try it anyway.

Since I started writing about my own cancer in *The Times* and other papers, I've had some 30,000 letters, of which about 5,000 have suggested alternative cures. About half of those letters talk of alternative cures that the writer or their friend or relation has undergone. Plenty of the letters use variants of the phrase 'And a year later he's still alive,' some use the phrase, 'Two years later she's still alive' and two of them used the phrase 'Three years later he's still alive.' I've yet to have a letter which includes the phrase 'Five (or ten or twenty) years later she's still alive' – although I've had plenty of mail from people who had orthodox treatment twenty or more years ago and are still around to write letters to newspaper columnists. As much to the point, I've yet to have a letter from a cancer patient who from the day of diagnosis eschewed orthodox treatment entirely in favour of one of the alternative versions, although I know that there are such.

The only reasonable deduction I can make from this is that all those people who took alternative therapies also took the orthodox ones and that none of them lived any longer than one might have expected as a result of using those alternative therapies.

So why are people so willing to believe these anecdotes about themselves and others, and pass them on? Again one can only guess, but there are enough narrative elements common to all or many of the stories to make the guess an educated one.

Most commonly there's the '. . . and the doctors couldn't believe it!' element. In fact, this has been a staple of the literature of Britons dealing with their doctors for years and it's a syndrome which includes such other equivalents as 'The doctor said he'd never seen one like it in all his working life.' We all like to believe in our uniqueness, which is reasonable enough, and never more so than when we're ill. And even if we're stoical about our own illnesses, we like to believe that the way our loved ones respond to treatment is some reflection on their essential goodness, inner strength or all-round superiority. When friends tell me that I must be some sort of medical marvel to have got this far with my cancer they're paying me a compliment: they're saying – however subconsciously – that I must be particularly strong or brave or clever or stoutly constitutioned to have lived four years after diagnosis when a year or two ago I told them that the cancer had gone terminal. What they've forgotten, of course, is that two years before that I was telling them that the cancer would be cured for good in a couple of weeks. And what they've not forgotten, because few of us really consider life in these terms, is that my survival this far isn't a matter of temperament or braveness, but of tiny chemical reactions over which I have no real control and over which my doctors have only slightly more. They can give me a drug in the knowledge that it has a 30 per cent chance of sending my cancer away for a while, but they can't – yet – give me a drug which has a 100 per cent chance of sending my cancer away for good.

Understandably, enough doctors conspire to utter this fraudulent currency along with the rest of us. Indeed, most of what passes as good bedside manner is various ways of allowing the sick to feel better about themselves, and that includes allowing them to believe that while in their healthy life they are ordinary, in sickness they are special. There have been plenty of times when my surgeon or my oncologist has strode into my ward after some test or another and announced, 'Fabulous results! Fabulous!' I'm sure they do it a dozen times a day, whenever they have to give news which isn't actually bad. Nobody has ever walked in with a batch of results and said, 'Absolutely ordinary. Just like most of the other patients!' For when they say 'fabulous', they're congratulating themselves on their superior skill, and me on my superior reaction to a drug or a scalpel cut, as if somebody who grows a cancer which is susceptible to surgery is in some way a better patient than some of their other patients who are stupid enough to grow their cancers too near to their carotid arteries for safety. It's a reasonable enough fiction: in this game there's not a lot which makes terminal patients feel good about themselves, and this is as good a result as any to cheer.

More, there comes a point in some illnesses when believing in the possibility of miracles is the only apparent option. And I'm not just talking about major or terminal illnesses where a miracle is the only possible difference between life and death. When he's lying in bed, wide awake at four in the morning, a patient with a chronically sore back which shows nothing that a doctor can get his hands on needs a miracle just as much as the cancer patient. It simply isn't any use hearing over and over in one's head, 'They said they couldn't find anything on the X-rays,' or, more frustrating still, 'They think I'm just imagining it.'

Paradoxically, though, miracles are in a statistical way much more possible than almost anything else.

Orthodox science, even at its hairier fringes, is based on a simple premise: that there is a set of laws which all scientific events obey. Some scientists think this set of laws is extremely small and are looking for that unified theory of everything; others think that the scientific book of laws is about the same size as the European Community's and that when it's finished those laws will line the walls of the scientific advocate like so many books on tort and contract.

But once you've discovered a law, the premise is that it applies for all conditions within its scientific jurisdiction. The second law of thermodynamics – the one about heat not passing from a colder to a hotter body – works all the time. That's why it's a *law* of thermodynamics, not a theorem. It turns out that in some cases there are different laws at a sub-molecular level, but within that jurisdiction they are still as all-encompassing.

And once you've established those laws, you establish a lot else about the way that matter – chemical, physical, biological – behaves even when that matter isn't an experimental ball-bearing hanging from a school lab's Newton's cradle.

Alternativism, though, posits that there are really no such laws. I can't tell you how many times I've been in debate with an alternativist when they've said of some physical impossibility, 'But how do you *know* it's not the case?', or 'But why are you so closed-minded that you won't believe that it happened just this time?', or, 'Yes, but what if in this case the stuff really did permeate the skin, for reasons we just don't understand?'

And this is the problem for people like me writing books like this. If you believe that science is a nonsense and that physics is a matter of random chance, then you can postulate anything. In order to demolish alternativism on the alternativist's terms I'd have to unpick every last 'what if?' and all those 'but perhaps just this once . . .'s. If I were a New Ager, though, who wanted to demolish the hundreds and thousands of rules and laws and working theories based on the assumption that to each action there is an equal and opposite reaction, then all I'd have to do is to show once – and conclusively – why this is wrong.

But there is another reason that people are prepared to accept passed-on stories as some sort of proof: often the people who pass them on aren't telling the truth. Don't get me wrong: I'm not saying that the purveyors of the examples I'm about to give are intentional liars – and no, this isn't just a way of getting round the legal problems of calling people liars in print; I really do believe that some of the factual myths which are perpetrated by believers in alternative therapies are held to be absolutely true. But it is the case that if I tell you a lie about a subject which you don't know a lot about, which doesn't look noticeably false, if my bona fides seem OK and I don't seem like the sort of person who would lie just for the hell of it, the chances are that you'd believe the odd untrue fact – even if I went on to build a whole structure of untruths based on the single false premise.

Take this statement, for instance: 'Scientists have no idea how aspirin works.'

Is that true or false? How could you tell – this side of looking it up in a medical library? In fact, it strikes me as just the sort of thing that might, oddly enough, be true. After all, aspirin has been used as such for just over a hundred years now, we know what it does and what its safety record is like – we don't actually *have* to know how it works in order to use it when we have a headache. In fact, I have no idea how most of the pills I take work, although I usually assume that someone at the drug company which made them does.

So if you heard somebody who seems to know what she's talking about – and seems to know more than you do on a subject – say that on a serious BBC radio discussion, you'd probably assume that it was true. I use it as an example because it was precisely what Lynne McTaggart of the *What Doctors Don't Tell You* newsletter and lobbying group said on a Radio Four discussion when she was debating with somebody from the Healthwatch organisation the wisdom of Middlesex University spending its money establishing a department to study Chinese traditional medicine.

In fact, to be accurate, she said, 'Scientists don't even know how aspirin works,' and the phrase was meant to suggest a) that orthodox medicine doesn't know as much as it pretends to and b) that traditional methodologies therefore have as much right to a slice of the research pie as any other.

Scientists don't know how aspirin works is one of those 'truths' which have been doing the rounds for years now and which, as it happens, just isn't true. Certainly for a long time medical science had only a basic idea of how non-steroidal-anti-inflammatory drugs (NSAIDs) like aspirin work, but since the middle of the last decade when researchers from the University of Chicago Medical Center published a paper on the subject, medical science has known precisely what happens when you take a couple of Alka-Seltzer. But when somone makes such a statement on a serious radio station, why should you not believe her?

Or take this quotation: '[Edgar Cayce] had the ability, while in a sleeping trance, to give absolutely accurate medical diagnoses and to prescribe totally appropriate treatments which used all available therapies. He successfully treated many thousands of patients, and despite many attempts to expose him, his reputation maintained complete integrity.'

That comes from *Holistic Revolution – the Essential New Age Reader* edited by William Bloom and published in 2000 by Allen Lane at the Penguin Press – a provenance I note not out of the usual publishing protocols but to point out that this is a serious book, properly published and, as I write, piled high at my local bookshop. Most people reading it, especially in Britain, where the Cayce cult never quite flourished as it did in the old fraud's homeland in the US, will have no reason (other than natural scepticism at the claims made for him in those forty-five words) to believe that Edgar Cayce's reputation maintained anything other than complete integrity: why should William Bloom – who has compiled a fascinating anthology and has himself an unimpeachable reputation in the field of holism – describe Cayce as such if it isn't the truth?

And yet even if you believe in the possibility that such sleeping trances are a possibility, you need to spend no more than a couple of minutes in a reasonably well-stocked library (or about forty-five seconds on the Net) to discover a hundred different ways in which Cayce's reputation maintained less than complete integrity even within his own lifetime. It's almost impossible to test the truth of the diagnosis-and-healing claims: they were all made by his followers and noted by his own amenuensis. It is, on the other hand, possible to test his claims that in 1958 the US would discover a form of death-ray used on the sunken island of Atlantis or his belief that in 1968 the Chinese would convert, en masse, to Christianity. This is not the place to argue the toss about Edgar Cayce; there are plenty of researchers who have written at length and critically on his activities. My point is not that there is or isn't some case to be made for Cayce, but that the bald statement that his reputation 'maintained complete integrity' can be passed on as truth merely by being stated so positively.

Some other medical 'facts' which are heaved about the place as if they were true include the following:

- More people die in American/British hospitals as a result of their treatment than of the disease they were admitted with.
- 80 (or, depending on who you're listening to, 90 or 95 per cent) of drugs used by orthodox doctors in Britain have never been formally tested under the conditions they demand for alternative remedies.
- Canadian hospitals have by law to offer Essiac treatment because this ancient Native American remedy has been shown to work.

None of these is true, all of them are provably false and in all three cases their roots can be traced from a sort of truth which was battered into submission over the years. Which looks, I know, as if I'm doing that which I promised I wouldn't do, and using an attack on alternativism to defend the orthodoxy. In fact, I'm pretty sure that many more people die of their treatment in hospital than is necessary and that all over the developed world doctors are happily doling out pre-scriptions for pharmaceutical drugs which are useless or next to it. But that isn't my point, which is that in order to make their case, the alternativists feel the need to use this sort of propaganda. If homeopathy worked, then it would be worth using regardless of whether hospital doctors are knowingly killing off their patients: it is patently safer, cheaper and has fewer side-effects than orthodox medicine.

Let me explain why.

OTHER PREOCCUPATIONS

15 MAY 1988

THE BLAND LEADING THE BLIND

IT'S A FUNNY old life here in the Flavour Squad. You plod on with your work – the routine stuff, handing out bad-taste tickets to another chain of pub steak houses taking liberties with the word *entrecôte*, giving a *final* final warning to the bloke who invented Angel Delight, dealing with an urgent monosodium glutamate call-out down at the local take-away, running an undercover stake-out at McDonald's, you know the sort of thing – when suddenly a case comes from out of nowhere which isn't covered by anything in Judges' Rules or Escoffier.

That's how it was with the yoghurt case. Or, as they call it down at the station, The Yoghurt Case. Of course, it had been going on for years; it was just that no one had noticed what was right under their noses. Until, that is, I reached into the station fridge for a yoghurt.

I'm a picky eater normally – well, you've got to be in my job – and the lads at the station have a bit of a chuckle about how I won't eat any yoghurt with mango or passion fruit in it. It never used to be a problem in the days when you knew the red ones were strawberry and the other red ones were raspberry, but these are strange times we live in. It had been a long shift and I'd only just got back from dragging some tinned bolognese sauce for soya-meat and so I just reached into the fridge, took the first pot that came to hand and ripped off the lid in one easy pull the way I learnt in my early days on Taste Patrol. Curse me for an impetuous fool, as the Super always says, but that's the way we are at the Flavour Squad.

85

I was about two spoonfuls in when it suddenly clicked: I didn't have the faintest idea what the yoghurt I was eating was trying to taste of.

It was a set yoghurt, with no fruit pulp to give it away, just a faint pink tinge which might have been evidence of a passing relationship with a strawberry or a raspberry or a stick of rhubarb or, knowing the fondness of the Chambourcy boys for fancy new flavours, Alpine radish or Albanian beetroot. And it wasn't as if the stuff was entirely flavourless under that cloying sweetness, just that the flavour wasn't a *real* flavour. Not what we at the Flavour Squad call a real flavour anyway.

It was just a hunch but with a hunch as strong as that there's hardly an eighteen-year-old Flavour Cadet around who wouldn't know what to do: a blind tasting. An identity parade we call it on the squad.

I staged a quick raid on a couple of chill cabinets and came away with thirty-eight pots of yoghurt. They were expert jobs from real masters: the St Ivel gang, the Boots boys up at Nottingham, the Chambourcys, of course, and the small Loseley outfit, who we've always found to be very upstanding when it comes to the flavour laws.

I quickly recruited three deputies (next-door neighbours but honest folk whose palates I'd trust in any rumble) and a referee. The ref covered up the pots with sticky paper, numbered each one and we started tasting. We did it according to the book: every spoon was washed between tastings, every mouth rinsed with mineral water, every sample properly smelt and held on the tongue for thirty seconds.

The hunch had been right. Out of the thirty-eight pots there were only two that all four of us could identify with certainty: Chambourcy Bonjour Lemon and Shape Rhubarb. The rest were all over the place.

The best guess-work was done by Julie, who got seventeen out of thirty-eight, but that was only by giving half a mark every time she made a stab at something like Fruits of the Forest and wrote down 'blackcurrant'.

Some of the yoghurts started off at a real disadvantage. There was no way anyone was going to identify Chambourcy's geranium or rosehip flavours and elderflower was listed either as 'watery apple' or 'oversweet vanilla' by all of us.

But we expected better of the straight flavours. The Chambourcy strawberry was tasted as 'something and lemon', 'apricot' and 'indescribable' by people who happily eat strawberry yoghurts every day. Two of us guessed Boots yoghurt to be strawberry (but not specifically Alpine Strawberry as per the label) but even a whole, small red fruit in my red Loseley live yoghurt didn't tell me I was eating their black cherry variety – it could have been a nude strawberry or a pallid blackcurrant or anything. Certainly it didn't taste of cherries and was listed variously as 'berry', 'unknown berry' and 'some sort of baby food – yuk' by the deputies. In fact, Loseley Very Low Fat Live came out of all this with a pretty bad record: the flavours were very dodgy and there's a chance that their texture will lead to a charge of impersonating a semolina with malicious intent.

But all that was nothing compared to the results we got from taking the multi-flavoured suspects to the interrogation room and giving them a seeing to. St Ivel Real Caribbean Fruits came out OK, but then even the station cat could probably suss out coconut and pineapple. As for the rest – Boots low-fat apple and blackberry was marked down as peach Melba on account of the shape of the lumps and the colour, Chambourcy peach and passion fruit was named as lychee.

We were in a bad state by the end, as would you be if you'd just turned over thirty-eight yoghurts. But we were all agreed: all yoghurts taste of sugar or sweetener and all flavourings are either so discreet as to be untasteable or so muddied as to be unrecognisable. Strawberry flavouring is a different flavour to strawberries, as is banana flavouring to bananas and chocolate flavouring to chocolate. But at least the flavourings are usually consistent: you can recognise strawberry flavouring for what it is whether you come across it in an instant milk shake or a packet jelly. Yoghurt's different, though. The colour and texture of a strawberry yoghurt is part of a conspiracy to make you believe what's written on the label. And you know what we think of conspiracy down at Flavour Patrol. Charges will be brought.

Now I know some of you consumerist do-gooders are going to say that all this is just a question of Flavour Patrol going in mob-handed where it's not needed. But next time you're passing the fridge, close your eyes, take out a yoghurt at random and see if *you* can guess the taste. Then ask yourself if you want your children to be brought up in the sort of society where flavour conspirators roam the supermarket shelves, preying on innocent young mouths. I think I know what the answer will be. Evening all.

Sunday Times Magazine

21 JANUARY 1989

GENEVA – FROM ROLEX TO OMEGA

CITIES ARE NEVER quite the stuff of their own mythology. Paris is full of Britons searching the Pigalle vainly for the ghost of Lautrec, London packed with Americans after fog and bobbies, Monte Carlo seethes with disappointed weekend sybarites in Moss Bros DJs.

Geneva, though: now there's a city which lives down to its expectations. All I expected of Geneva was banks and wrist watches. Banks and wrist watches were just what I got.

My friend, who spends whole weeks at a time in Geneva doing something valiant for the Red Cross, says that Geneva is all those things that those fanatical about any city say their city is. A city of contrasts, a city of towering this and subterranean that and cosmopolitan the other. Name a city you *haven't* heard that about.

The contrasts in Geneva are between light grey and dark, between affluent and well-off, between Rolex and Omega. The cathedral towers, but with a backdrop of 180-degree alp a cathedral has to do an awful lot of towering to make its point.

There is, says my friend, a bohemian quarter, Carouge, a sort of Genevois Amsterdam. My friend obviously thinks a couple of lines of desultory graffiti and the odd fly-posted advertisement make for bohemianism, but this is the town of Calvin and Knox, where the most modest of rebellions counts as a manifesto.

Compromise rather than revolution is the stuff of Geneva: outside the old town it is the province of the UN and the ILO and the ICRC and any number of other acronymous organisations which fill the large, flat-sided buildings with oratorical inaction.

People do not make waves in Geneva; the banks least of all. Whole streets in the centre of town go bank, Rolex, bank, bank, Patek Philippe, bank, bank, Japanese electronics store, bank, bank, bank, Longines, greengrocer, Omega, bank, bank, bank. The tops of buildings sprout giant neon signs bearing the names of watch companies and banks, the way other European cities have signs for cigarettes and beer. The rue du Rhône, the main shopping street, is a couple of Benettons, a few Inter-Chics and about three dozen branches of Bally.

At the airport the car rental company rep wouldn't let me speak French ('I have not the time, sir'), took the retail price of a small hatchback off me for a couple of days' hire, and suggested that I stay at the Metropole. This would, he said happily, cost me an arm. Presumably there are other hotels which charge the leg too.

I could afford an arm. After all, the idea was to motor down to a conference I had to attend in Montreux, staying in the Swiss equivalent of the cheap *pensions* which every village across the lake in France has. Had I known that the *pension* is an unknown concept in Switzerland I might have gone for somewhere more modest in Geneva. An ear's worth, perhaps.

The Metropole is, says the sign in the Michelin, a grand hotel. In reality they play at grand hotels there, and their unconvincing bowing and scraping does not make up for small rooms, surly room service or packet food for room-service meals. Never mind: I had a view over the lake and my balcony overlooked the lake and my balcony overlooked the Rade. At least, I assume it was the Rade: my friend described the fountain as the sort of thing people cross continents to see. I saw a small piddling thing with a central spume knocked off-centre by a quite gentle breeze.

I should have been able to predict my disappointment, after all the stuff about contrast and beauty and cosmopolitanism. My friend had paid Geneva the two greatest compliments he could think of. The first was that the airport was terribly close to the city, the second that Hergé, in one of his books, had put Tintin into the city's best hotel.

The next morning I waited half an hour for the mist to clear the lake and then gave up and went to buy a watch.

Swiss watches used to be solid things, instruments of, at best, discretion, at worst substance. Since quartz movements dispossessed the Swiss horologists of their advantage of accuracy they have gone instead for gaudiness. Watches drip with tiny diamonds, curl in unattractive golden sweeps around the plastic wrists in the window displays, or bear dials crammed with as many smaller dials as will fit on. There are lumbering great ingots of gold with which a man may break his wrist trying to tell the time, compact little wrist-sculptures with which his wife may go blind trying to read the hands. All of them, cheap quartz Swatches included, cost every bit as much as they do in London.

So I had a steak (I can't bring myself to eat fondue in London so I see no reason why I should do so in Geneva), decided it was raining too hard to take one of the commuter boats which criss-cross the lake, and set off to find my *pension*.

There are two routes around the lake: the pretty one and the motorway. (There is also the train, which my friend says is scenic in the extreme, but I had given up on his discrimination in such matters and anyway I had the car.) The pretty route manages to miss much of the lake for the first part of its length, but when I hit Vaud proper (Vaud is the semi-rural canton where the Genevois live now that the delegate level has risen to 40 per cent of the city's population and sent property prices alp-high) the mist cleared, the road lifted and there it was with the mountains rising behind it.

There are three things to see in the anodyne Vaud landscape: cyclists, mopedists and big, sad-eyed, snuff-brown cows. Which is not to say the drive lacked a certain excitement, given that the highway code in Switzerland seems to be a voluntary affair. In a country where Geneva, the most sophisticated and cosmopolitan city, shuts tight at midnight, the locals get their kicks by overtaking on blind corners.

I was beginning to worry about somewhere to stay. I had

run out of arms and the pretty lakeside hotel in Coppet wanted another one for a room. I tried one of the slab-sided, grey chateaux that lowered above the road but it was closed. The next town was closed for a wedding, the next to that closed just for the fun of it. I drove up hill and down dale in a canton whose long suit is hills and dales, and eventually found Mex and l'Auberge au Mai.

The *patron* hummed and hahed and eventually lent me one of his five empty guest rooms for sixty francs, gave me another steak ('*Fondue, monsieur? Pas de fondue, monsieur*') and suggested I walk around.

Mex at night-time is everything Heidi would have wanted from a village. An ancient town hall with a wooden châlet roof dropping to head height, a square old college building (converted into flats for the Genevois refugees), a steeply pitched Calvinist church and the feel of an over-preserved Cotswold village. Mex under Stour, Mex over Wychwood, something like that.

I got back to the *auberge* to find a wedding party in progress. They closed the door on the wedding room as I passed and so I took a glass of sour Vaud wine to bed.

At midnight a silver band came to play for the wedding. At one it was replaced by a gramophone. At two they all began to sing along. At three, when they all began to play a game which apparently involved running up and down bare boards in clogs while beating zinc pails with soup ladles and screaming, I went down to complain. '*Monsieur, je suis désolé. Désolé*,' said the *patron*, who had forgotten he had a resident that night.

At seven he returned, still *désolé* and hungover with it, and presented me with a cup of coffee by way of apology, and at eight I drove to Lausanne. My *Guide Bleu* gives six pages to Lausanne, which by my reckoning is five too many. Both the cathedral and the church of St François were closed, and the surrounding greyness made Geneva look Technicolor by comparison.

But driving back to the lake road, there was Ouchy, which, says the *Guide*, I could have ridden down to in a funicular. Ouchy is as splendid a little resort as any you will find inland anywhere. It has nothing to do with its Britishness (English church, Hotel d'Angleterre, late residence of Byron and Shelley, and where Byron knocked off the 'Prisoner of Chillon' in forty-eight hours flat) but with the lake. So far the lake had been an adjunct to its towns and villages. At Ouchy it is part of the town. The hotels and bars and cafés cluster round it, restaurants pitch themselves over it, the lake buzzes with yachts and little motor boats.

That night I finally reached Montreux, found that my conference was yet to start, that my hotel, the Bonivard, was a mile west of town and that most of the flashier restaurants were booked solid.

So I went to Harry's American Bar, ordered four large whiskies, drove drunkenly (but still in a straighter line than the horribly sober locals) back to the hotel, and slept through the first conference session.

Two days later I drove back to Geneva airport. I took the motorway.

Spectator

10 JUNE 1989

WATER, WATER EVERY WAY

WHEN THE TIME comes to undertake that most tedious of tasks, the preparation of the social history of the 1980s, I would direct historians not to the Public Records Office, but to the inventory computer of the Tesco superstore which sits on the wrong side of Rotherhithe in south London. (There is perhaps more than enough social history revealed in the fact that Rotherhithe now has a *right* side, but no matter.)

From this record we shall learn that by mid-1989 Tesco's, the least style-conscious of all supermarket chains, in Rotherhithe, the least upwardly-mobile of all London's docklands, stocked sixteen separate varieties of bottled water. Add to those varieties the sub-species of French water with a twist of lemon and Scottish water with a hint of lime, and the range of waters from which Rotherhithe's superannuated dockers have to choose rises to some twenty-five.

Who *needs* twenty-five brands of water? True, we once needed bottled water in France because we could never quite trust the *eau municipale* and we needed Malvern water to give whisky and water a consistency of taste throughout the country. But where in Rotherhithe is the market for Ramlösa Carbonated Natural Mineral Water from the Source Ramlösa Brunn in Sweden? Or for Ballygowan Non-sparkling Natural Irish Spring Water from County Limerick? How do we know that the Source Ramlösa Brunn is not the local name for Malmo's main sewage outflow? How many Rotherhithe palates, honed on Worthington India Pale Ale can distinguish

Chiltern Hills Water from Buxton Spring Water? More to the point, why would they want to?

Bottled water is no longer an exercise in hygiene or even in taste, but in marketing, and the marketed image of every brand is exactly the same. The key word on almost every bottle is natural. (On the French bottles they say *naturelle*, but I'm told this means much the same.) The implication here is that somewhere, in a lock-up garage in Fulham, is some Arthur Daley character craftily bolting a couple of hydrogen atoms on to one of oxygen to produce dodgy artificial water which might *taste* the same but in some imperceptible way is a lesser water.

The second come-on is the table of contents. By tradition French waters have always been labelled with a chart showing the precise amount of sodium, chlorides, sulphates and so on as adduced by the official analyst in 1921 (or whenever). This is only reasonable: it is worth knowing that Volvic has calcium 10.4 mg/l and nitrates 4 mg/l in a country where in 1921 the stuff from the tap usually contained cattle slurry 104 mg/1 and Charlemagne's Revenge 265 mg/l. To know that Highland Spring Water had a conductivity in 1985 of 255, in a country where tap water has a conductivity of 255 does not mean a great deal.

Stranger still is the fact that some of the constituent 'natural' chemicals which figure so proudly in these analyses are the same chemicals which the modern cardio-conscious set (the sort at which these waters are pitched) are warned to be wary of. A high sodium content might have been thought fine when the French analyses were made in the Twenties; now we know better.

There are other ploys which are more facile still. Spa mineral water from Belgium is, says the can, 'The ideal thirst quencher'. Well, of course it's the ideal thirst quencher: it's water. That's what water does, for God's sake: it quenches thirst.

Highland Spring, according to its label, is 'Calorie Free', unlike, I take it, all those fatty waters you see about the place. And here's another tip: when drinking Badoit, it is best served chilled. Chilled water, eh? Bet the Badoit food economists were up all night working that one out. It must have come to them at around the same time as the idea that as well as being 'the perfect accompaniment to good food and fine wines' it can even be served 'as a refreshing drink in its own right'. Chiltern Hills water takes the recipe line further: why not add it to fruit cordials or drink it with a slice of lemon? What, you mean like you can with water?

The biggest deal about all bottled water is 'the source'. All waters need a 'source' to sell themselves ever since the Source Perrier became a tourist attraction in its own right. On the Volvic bottle, therefore, we have a diagrammatic representation of the source: this stratum is basalt, that granite, the other *surface humus* or, as we say on *Gardeners' Question Time*, a humus surface. Chiltern Water, says the bottle, spends fifty years seeping through a ninety-million-year-old chalk stratum.

What this means is that God and the Thames Water Authority agree that the best way of purifying water is to pass it through porous rock. It is just that when the water board does the job it uses progressively fine sand and other silicates many at least ninety million years old.

There is nothing which says that a water purified by Chiltern rock is going to be any purer, tastier, safer or healthier than water purified by Southend sand. Aqua Pura from Church Stretton, Shropshire, makes such claims only by implication. 'The source lies at the foot of the Long Mynd, an area rich in Roman History and now protected by the National Trust.' What sort of recommendation is this meant to be? The Thames at Reading runs through an area rich in Roman history and protected by the National Trust, but I wouldn't drink the water from it.

Last year British sales of bottled water – at recommended retail as opposed to £1-a-glass restaurant prices – hit £216 million. The irony: as the water boards start advertising themselves as purveyors of pure H_2O to the masses, we have become apparently so worried about what actually happens out of the tap that we are happy to buy any bottled water as long as it has got a pretty picture of a French (or Scottish or Irish) mountain on the label.

Never mind the fact that some parts of the country drink,

for free, precisely the same chalk-filtered stuff as they buy in Tesco's. And never mind, either, that the price of Buxton water which flows from the spring in Derbyshire is, at 59p per litre, rather more expensive than the heavily-taxed, highly refined petrol which is hard won from the raging North Sea.

What is truly surprising is not that the Golf GTi and mobile phone set have fallen for this water malarkey, but that Rotherhithe's yeoman stock, who you would have thought would have known better than to pay £2.50 a gallon for water, are queueing up for the stuff.

Spectator

28 JULY 1990

CUTTING A WOODEN DASH

'WHAT I WANT to know,' said a recent correspondent of one of the dozen or so old car magazines, 'is whether my 1976 Ford Capri is a classic car yet or not.'

Imagine writing to *Decanter* magazine and asking whether it's worth bunging a dozen of the 1990 Babycham in the cellar next to the '45 Petrus, and you have the picture. Especially if you go on to imagine *Decanter* suggesting that given a couple of years in the bottle the Babycham will turn into a fine, if unassuming little drink, well worth the modest investment.

Until a decade ago there were two main markets for used cars. One was called Vintage and Veteran and involved men in window-pane-check plus-fours burnishing the brass ignition advance levers of old Lagondas. The other was called Honest Trev's Used Cortinarama and involved men in window-pane-check Burton's suits sticking ignition advance springs back on with Araldite.

There was, as well, a third and insignificant market which used to be called Clapped-out-old-bangers and involved men in greasy overalls hitting the ignition with a lead mallet. It is that third market which has evolved into the modern classic car industry.

Definition: a modern classic car is any car about which someone under fifty has ever tutted fondly and said, 'My God! Look at that! I had one of those in 1968. My first car, that was: cost me twenty-five quid and I had to break an egg into the radiator once a week to stop it leaking.'

Thus the Sunbeam Alpine is a classic car. The Rover P6 is a

classic car. According to the members of the Hillman Avenger Club, the Hillman Avenger is, for God's sake, a classic car. Remember the Avenger? An underpowered mélange of scrap metal and cardboard cogs and the nearest thing to canine life that ever limped out of Coventry. Well, now it's a classic.

'Classic' in this context does not have anything to do with purity of form: the purity of a Triumph TR8's form is negligible, but one with its original go-faster stripes in place will fetch £7,000 on a good day. Classic simply means any car that doesn't look like one of the Eurojap tin boxes which pass for the modern car. A car of which to say, 'Can't imagine a Fiesta lasting twenty years, can you?' as you put your foot hard down on the throttle and go through the rusted floor-pan on the follow-through.

Real classic cars are those which had their own sense of posterity hand-built into them on an engineer's bench. Modern classics are those which had their own sense of chassis-rot screwed into them on a production line in Birmingham but which somehow have lasted through the decades.

Classic – ancient and modern – also means investment. Investment cars used to mean a Bugatti bid for at Christie's or a Lagonda bought from a mews garage in Kensington. Then it came to mean a refurbished E-Type, a postwar drop-head with a dicky seat, or any car where the right chassis number was a selling point. But with good E-Types regularly fetching £100,000 and more, and ten-year-old major-league Ferraris selling at a quarter of a million, the market began to get a bit tight. Old cars had a cachet, but too much of a price for the driver looking for an alternative to his company Montego.

And just as the price of old Alvises and Facel Vegas trebled and quadrupled over the past five years, so, hopes the man who has just bought his tatty fifteen-year-old MG, will the price of the modern classic.

There are, perhaps, half-a-dozen categories of modern classic to choose from. There are, for instance, all those mass-market substitutes for thoroughbreds. The Volkswagen Karmann Ghia, for instance, was always a bit of a joke in its day when it was seen as a sort of fake, latter-day Panhard. Now you'll hear enthusiasts discussing its shared Porsche lineage – and this despite sharing a noisy air-cooled engine with the Beetle. A restored convertible costs around £10,000; a restorable fixed-head around £4,000 – usually complete with rotting bodywork. The Volvo P1800 – the car Roger Moore used to drive as the Saint – works on the same squat, cartoon-sports-car principle: about £3,000 buys a good version, £6,000 one in the very best condition.

Then there are the sportyish pocket-tourers with which the big Midlands manufacturers augmented their range of family cars in the Sixties and Seventies. There are those, for instance, who say that the Triumph Spitfire is something more than a Herald with a poncy body, but then there are those who say that Rome is the capital of France. Any of the sporty MG and Triumph coupés now counts as a classic: in order of desirability they go something like TR2, TR3, TR4, MGA, TR6, MGB V8, MGB, GT6, Midget, Spitfire, TR7. Prices range from £18,000 for the best TRs to £1,800 for an ordinary version of anything below an MGB.

The alternatives are marques which are even longer dead than Triumph and MG. (No, the MG Metro does *not* count – any more than an Austin-Healey Escort.) The sportier open-top Sunbeams are reckoned cars: Alpines are still cheap, but Tigers are ludicrously expensive.

In fact, any old convertible fetches a price now that the common consensus is that, with the top sliced off the ozone layer, it's a matter of weeks before residents of Cap Ferrat start coming over to Watford to top up their tans.

The rag-top version of the Herald-Vitesse range is the car about which dealers are currently saying, 'Can't let that go for under four grand, squire – two years from now and you're looking at ten grand, easy.' Which is what they once said about the Stag, and they were right.

A Vitesse has a two-litre, six-pot engine, the turning circle of a London taxi, looks good on women who drive with the top down while wearing a leopard-print headscarf and dark glasses, and costs under £6,000 for a pristine example. They will cost more. (I hope so, at least: your restaurant critic has just bought one to go with her leopard-print headscarf for £3,000.)

Spectator

1 December 1990

ABDICATION SPECIAL

THE BEST CAMPAIGN of all was run by Mrs Emma Nicholson. 'It's a rather fascinating new game,' she told *Channel 4 News* on the night of the abdication. The game, as played so consummately by Mrs Nicholson, was this:

1   Tease media on Thursday with the announcement that while you support Mrs Thatcher, your constituents might just persuade you to change your mind.

2   Return on Friday to say that you promise to tell the cameras what you're doing on Monday, so guaranteeing another turn in front of them after the weekend.

3   Announce on Monday that you're coming out for Heseltine, thus becoming the backbencher all the producers go for when they want the word from the backbencher who has changed sides.

By the time the nominations were in for the second round Mrs Nicholson had managed, by my reckoning, eight goes in front of the camera and it can only be a matter of time before she sells the rights of her game to Waddington's: Stab in the Back, a jolly board game for one to 372 players.

Once the announcement came it was all rather anticlimactic. The BBC went for the catch-all 'Maggie Under Bus' contingency plan and ran what seemed to be straight obituary footage with Margaret looking about thirty-five and Denis looking sober; ITV tried some mild political commentary. Either way I tallied the *in memoriam* content as: 1973 'There will never be a woman prime minister in my lifetime' footage: seven times; 1974 winter of discontent black plastic bags and unfilled graves montage: eight times; 1979 Number 10 Francis of Assisi speech: ten times; 1983 'Rejoice! Rejoice!' message: five times; 1981 party conference 'This lady's not for turning' speech: nine times; sundry pictures of yuppies popping champagne, youngsters dossing in cardboard boxes, shirt-sleeved brokers frowning at flickering City computer screens, Arthur Scargill looking mock-noble at the head of a column of pitmen, memorial plaque at Grantham High School (weeping sixth-former: 'We all look up to her – she's our role model'), Argentinian battleship sinking: 187 times.

None of which explained quite why the abdication had taken place, but then by Sunday when the heavyweight political shows were putting the three prime ministers-in-waiting through their paces, it didn't really matter very much.

'The day when politics is completely dominated by images is the day when it goes completely downhill,' Douglas Hurd told Jonathan Dimbleby, which given that he'd spent the previous five minutes trying to create the unlikely image of himself as a horny-handed son of toil ('I had to plant the potatoes fifteen inches apart at ninepence a day') rang just a little hollow. While Walden did his standard impression of Uncle Brian the Statesman's Chum, Dimbleby spent his time putting down a pettish marker for the prime ministerial interviews to come.

The result was less than illuminating. All three agreed that the other two were really terribly capable chaps who might well do the job just as well as the interviewee himself would. Pressed (or, in Walden's case, massaged with sweet-smelling oil), John Major said that the campaign was about choice, Michael Heseltine that it was about getting the poll tax right and Douglas Hurd that he was sure he'd get a good novel out of it all some day. *House of Cards Revisited*, perhaps?

Spectator

22 December 1990

ANYONE CAN BE A WORDSMITH

Mr E. H. Metcalfe has written from Manchester to tell me that, if I send him £189, 'The world can literally be your oyster.'

A test then:

i) Does E. H. Metcalfe know what the word 'literally' means?

ii) Does E. H. Metcalfe know what an oyster looks like?

iii) What do you think are the chances of my becoming a well-paid and successful writer under Mr Metcalfe's tutelage?

Mr Metcalfe is principal of the Writers Bureau (no, I don't know what's happened to the possessive apostrophe either) of Dale Street, Manchester. You will have seen his advertisements in the quality press or, if not his, then those of the London School of Journalism, the Writing School, or the David and Charles Writers' College.

All offer to get you into print as a journalist, novelist, playwright or poet. Or, as one of the postal academies – Wallace Arnold's alma mater I'd vouchsafe – has it, a wordsmith.

The thing is, you see, that anyone can be a writer. You thought Bernard Levin or Keith Waterhouse got where they are today by habitually choosing the right word and then slotting it in there in the right place? That's just what the writers' mafia would *have* you believe.

For what these smug initiates will never tell you, and what only plucky Judy Chard, Director of Studies of the David and Charles Writers' College, is willing to come right out and say, is that 'You already know several thousand words and you are able to put them together every time you talk.' Well, perhaps not *every* time, Miss Chard, but I take your point.

It's those several thousand words which are the secret. Pick a few of the right ones and you're halfway there. To get all the way there, simply commit to memory a number of dodges which would ensure those million donkeys with their typewriters would *all* end up writing *Hamlet*.

There are, for instance, the Writing School's Six Rules for Evolving Plots and the Four Rules for Strengthening Plots. The Writers Bureau offers its failsafe Plot Planner and Subject Analyser, and the David and Charles Writers' College has its Television Action Digest.

I was tempted. Which writer, deadline long gone and whisky bottle down to the dregs, hasn't wanted some sort of literary ready-reckoner that will turn a plotless ramble into vintage Maugham? But ask yourself: would you buy a used novel from whoever wrote this synopsis of the 'More About Characterisation' lesson of the Writing School's course? I give it to you precisely as it was given to me:

'Your study moves on to the techniques of presenting emotion through your Characters . . . how your Characters can show fear, anxiety, anger, jealousy, shyness, happiness – and of course Love. Writing the Love Scene is an important skill to develop because of the scope for interreaction between your Characters. You learn how to characterise the Heroine, the Hero, the Villain – by writing-in their major and minor emotional traits. You see how to express Character in Dialogue, discover how Characterisation harnesses Human Behaviour Patterns and Motivation. Perhaps most fascinating of all you learn how to observe character traits in the people you meet every day, and how to create Characters from experience.' Heavy on the shift key, or what? Or maybe the rules of capitalisation come after the Love Scene in the syllabus.

The Writing School's prospectus for its course – 'most attractively presented in a library sleeve which will grace any bookshelf' – reads like a series of penny novelette chapter headings: 'An important truth for all writers – deciding where and when to write – a danger to avoid – advice from Arnold

Bennett', through to 'H. G. Wells' method for success – how to use rejections to improve your writing – how to keep yourself at your mental peak – essential advice from Lord Northcliffe . . . how to avoid sounding arrogant – the dangers of sentimentality'.

But persevere. 'The most important quality you require is not brilliance, but perseverence' (sic) confides Mr Metcalfe, and eventually the literal thing with the oysters will start to happen. 'I have sold another short story bringing my earnings to £291. I shall always be grateful to the Writing School for making my small dream come true,' enthuses Mrs ME from Essex in that school's come-on pack. A small dream indeed. MH of Manchester adds, 'I have managed to sell three articles and a short story totally £91 in payment.' At £23 a knob, I only hope MH is working hard at his day job. £23 for even the shortest story is not a fortune, not even a small one. A thousand words sold to any national newspaper would have doubled MH's earnings for four pieces, a single short piece in any good colour supplement trebled them.

But then the Writers Bureau's list of past successes suggests that MH would never have aimed quite that high: '"Conker Time" has been accepted for publication by the *Lady*,' says a grateful Sylvia Wade and, 'The satirical article that I wrote for assignment 2 was accepted by the *Truth* magazine' boasts Michael Hopkins. Alan Johnson managed to get 'A Spade is a Spade' into *Amateur Gardening*, and Writing School graduate DG of Penrith has 'won £117 worth of camping equipment by writing a slogan following the example of one of the School books sent with the Writing School course.' Yes, I know Hemingway started somewhere too, but it wasn't by writing tie-breakers for camping competitions.

But then in a down-page burst of candour, Judy Chard doubts 'if you will become a household name – only a few writers in every generation have that much talent – nor will you become rich and famous'. Fame, of course, isn't the only spur: 'Achieve instant success! See your name in print like Mr Priest of Barmouth,' shrieks the David and Charles Writers' College and, more modestly, 'It was quite exciting to see something I had written in print,' says Writers Bureau graduate John Lockley. The general consensus is that no true artist minds starving when he can send a copy of *Cage and Aviary Birds* with his byline on it to his mum.

There is, of course, nothing wrong with writing for *Prediction* or *Loving* or *Mother* or any of the other waiting-room magazines, and if they pay pin-money then, the NUJ notwithstanding, that's what they pay. But a 1,500-word article, 'Foxes, Farms and Fossils', as sold to *Dorset Life* by GW of that county doth not an income make. And given that Saturday and Sunday papers are screaming for copy to fill their gaping, multi-supplemental maws, and will pay the fillers top rate for helping out with the rush, why should a budding writer not look further than 'a letter to *Titbits* for which I received £20 (GL, Scotland)'?

Perhaps it's because the one point that none of these brochures makes is that although the quality press is full of well-paid-for freelance articles, hardly any of them were submitted speculatively. Certainly, in a dozen years as a full-time journalist I've never written a word without getting an agreement from an editor that it will be paid for and published.

To that extent the freelance journalism business is unfair: I have spent long hours turning commissioned and sub-literate copy from household-name journalists into something that stands a chance of getting read, and then minutes writing rejection slips to competent amateurs who have sent in entirely readable, but unwanted and unsuitable, pieces on spec.

I could always spot, by the way, a correspondence writing school graduate's efforts. It always came with a neatly folded manila SAE for its return and a brisk letter which begged the 'favour of consideration'. It would be Amstrad word-processed in neat double-spacing, and a paragraph would never be allowed to turn a page. At the bottom of each folio would be the word *More* – very professional that – and at the end of the last was the hopefully arrogant annotation 'First British Rights only © Trelawney O'Wells 1990'. Like a school project book whose author hopes that fancy presentation will serve as a decoy from lousy contents, blank, save for an improbably alliterative title like 'Cats, Craters and Catamites'.

Why does speculative writing so rarely get published by the big payers? Partly for the masonic reasons you'd suspect: old pals commissioning each other, editors feeling safer with a name they know, minor acts of blackmail, free lunches being paid for. But it's mainly because writing is a business like any other, and editors feel much the same about part-time dilettantes as policemen feel about Neighbourhood Watch schemes.

None of which is to say that amateurs can't become part- or full-time professionals. After all, I did once. But if you can write (and if, like most people, you can't, no correspondence course will help you), then it should be possible to condense all you need to know about getting your work published into two sheets of A4 paper.

And no, since you ask, I won't send you those two sheets. Not without a commissioning note, anyway.

Spectator

MAY 1991

HOW MEN SIZE UP THE OPPOSITION

BEFORE A PILOT taxies up the runway, he does a pre-flight check with his co-pilot. You know the sort of thing: 'Ailerons down?' the pilot says. 'Ailerons down,' the co-pilot repeats. 'Flaps up? Fuel tanks full? Yesterday's in-flight dinners scraped off the portholes?' And the co-pilot checks the flaps, fuel gauge and portholes and repeats the mantra.

Well, I used to have a girlfriend like that. We'd dress to go out: 'Lipstick straight?' Lipstick straight. 'Dress not too long?' Nope, dress not too long. 'Too short then?' Nor too short. 'The top doesn't make me look fat, does it?' Darling, it doesn't make you look fat.

I wouldn't mind, but this was for a trip to the supermarket. And then, over the months, the pre-Tesco flight check got longer. 'Is my face slightly fatter than it was last week? And those bags under my eyes – do they make me look five years older? Be honest. What do you *mean*, they do? My God! I've just seen myself in the mirror! How can you let me go out looking like this?'

By the time we'd had the argument about whether I could find a way of responding which didn't involve grinding my teeth down to my gums, the film had started or the party was over; and this is why I speak of this girlfriend in the past tense. But this is not the preamble to the standard male huh!-women-they-take-over-five-hours-to-get-ready-and-then-complain-all-night-that-they've-got-mismatched-stockings rant, but an admission. And the admission is: I'm just the same. It's not that much of an admission. All men are the same, they just pretend they're not.

Every so often I will be sitting in a bar with a woman, and a man will pass. A good-looking man, firm of jaw and tight of bottom. He will be dressed more elegantly than I am and the bartenders will rush to serve him. The woman will turn to me and say, 'That guy, do you think he's attractive?'

Now, every man knows that when a woman says that, what she means is, 'I'd like to ogle that bloke for a few minutes and the only way I can do it without you becoming boringly jealous is to turn this into an academic discussion on the nature of male beauty.' And what men come back with is, 'Don't ask me – what do I know about what makes a man attractive to women?' This, however, is nothing more than a bit of hasty camouflage for the average man's feelings of inadequacy. Every man has read the tabloid surveys which show that women are turned on by – in order of preference – a tight bottom, a good head of hair, a fair-sized set of pecs and a full wallet. Equally, every man knows the difference between a tight bottom and the slack and wobbly item seen on darts players. But, somewhere in the back of his psyche, every man (and you can assume that the word 'heterosexual' attaches to all men herein described) fears that to recognise a tight bottom means that he has designs on it. And by 'design' I don't mean a tattoo of Madonna.

It's much the same when men get together. Every so often a glossy magazine will run a piece which says that this is the year of the male cosmetic. Trust me on this one: it isn't. One reason that a woman has no problem buying make-up is that, however intellectually gifted she may be, she feels that a discussion on the difference between Lancôme's Niosôme and Arden's Immunage is a reasonable way of passing a spare five minutes. But I cannot foresee a day in my lifetime when one man will say to another, 'You know, Ted, this new Barry Sheen lipgloss stays on for hours and, after a day in the steelworks, that's a real boon.' Saying that would be stating, by implication, what every woman states when she looks in a make-up mirror: 'You know, Ted, I don't really like the way I look. I wish my eyes were bigger and my lashes longer. I'd like redder cheeks, fuller lips and smoother skin.'

109

The proof can be seen in any barber's shop. Women go into their hairdresser's with pages torn from *Hairdressing Weekly*, point to a picture and say, 'Look, I want you to tint it the colour of Michelle Pfeiffer, give it the body of Rula Lenska and the length of Cher.' The woman is simply acknowledging that she makes some sort of visual impression and that this impression is capable of improvement. A man, on the other hand, will go to his barber and say, 'Same as last time,' and hope that he doesn't look too much like Norman Wisdom when he leaves. At most, he may ask the barber what he thinks in the fervent hope that the barber will say something like, 'Well, it's always struck me that you have something of the Ted Danson about you. How about we darken it a little and then build up the front . . .' And the man will say, 'Sounds like a lot of fuss to me, but you're the expert,' and thus distance himself from the actual act of considering his looks.

I have a friend who split up with his wife a few years ago. The first thing he did was grow a small pigtail. 'Hey, Charles! Love the pigtail!' I said, and meant it. It gave him a certain sort of 1986 rakishness. 'Oh, that,' he said. 'Well, the hair was getting a bit long and I sort of cut it myself and the pigtail just got left behind.' Even if the lock of hair hadn't been bound by a new and very elaborate leather braid, that was palpable rubbish: Charles fancied himself as a pigtail wearer but wasn't saying so.

The point is this: for a man to acknowledge his haircut or the shape of his face is to suggest that his attractiveness is vested in something other than an innate and abstract maleness. Look at the paunchy and balding brickie wolf-whistling passing girls, or the oleaginous middle manager leching his way around the typing pool: somewhere within them they both believe that they are competing – and believe me they do see it as a competition – on equal terms with their intended prey. It is *because* men – however boorish, unattractive, ill-kempt or stupid they are – maintain the belief that their unassailable trump card lies comfortably in the pouch of their Y-fronts that they are uptight when called upon to consider attractiveness, or otherwise, of their own sex. There are exceptions, of course, but phoney exceptions. Body builders will discuss their biceps and triceps with each other, but their discussion is couched in academic terms. They will say, 'I've been doing this new pec curl and it's put over 1.2mm on the muscle,' when what they really mean is, 'Hey, sucker – look at these arms and weep.'

And there are times when men are so mystified by the sexual magnetism of one of their fellows that they're willing to hazard a question or two about it. I must have had the, 'But precisely what *is* it that you find so attractive about John Thaw?' conversation some half a dozen times since *Inspector Morse* first appeared. And, when a woman at a dinner party last week listed for the amazed assembly the things she would gladly do with John Major between a pair of black satin sheets, it was the men at the table who demanded the details of the Great Grey One's allure.

The Catch-22 of the male self-image is that, while it's cool to look good, it's uncool to want to look good. And all those male insults: 'He's a snappy dresser,' might sound like a compliment, but it's nothing of the sort. And a man forced to acknowledge the looks of some notoriously handsome actor will usually describe him as 'a good-looking bastard', as if being obviously attractive is cheating. But when it comes down to it, I suppose it's not that we want to look handsome, but that we want all other men to look ugly.

She

111

6 FEBRUARY 1992

THE FIRST DATE: MAKING

IT WATERTIGHT

As IF SEDUCTION wasn't already hard enough, an American lawyer has devised a legal form for both parties to sign before a first date. I'd guess that the document is no more than a series of get out clauses should the date end in pregnancy or a blood test, but I doubt whether that's quite the sort of contract we need in this country. Aids and unmarried motherhood might be a worry for some, but it's the smaller courtesies of first dating that really need to be legally addressed . . .

A Contract between Henry Cripps (hereinafter to be known as The Dater) and Caroline Bastaple (hereinafter to be known as The Datee).

1: Notwithstanding the Arsenal match being postponed, the penultimate episode of Moon and Son being a bit of a cliffhanger, or a last-minute pick-up at the Two Horseshoes after work on Friday, The Dater and The Datee agree to meet at the Omar Khayyam Tandoori Centre, Ealing W5, at 8.30pm on Saturday (hereinafter referred to as The Date) always allowing that The Datee may be no more than 20 (twenty) and no less than 10 (ten) minutes later without incurring penalties under rider 3(i): Emotional blackmail.

2: It is hereby understood that in that The Date shall take place in order that The Dater may discuss a couple of really quite interesting ideas he's got for the marketing meeting on Tuesday on which he'd like some creative input from The Datee, both parties shall terminate such discussion no later than 3 (three) minutes after the onion bhajis have been served. At this point both parties shall undertake to determine from each other:

112

i: Whether The Dater is still seeing Jennifer from Accounts Pending (hereinafter referred to as A Bit Tarty If You Ask Me, But Then Some Men Go For The Obvious Type);

ii: Whether The Datee really stung that fool Nigel in Corporate Holdings for a five-course meal at Luigi's, plus entrance to Stringfellows including six large Drambuie and Cokes, plus a cab home and then gave him a kiss on the cheek and left him standing on the doorstep';

iii: How The Dater recalls the very first time he saw The Datee across the photocopying room and even though they didn't speak until the Christmas party, he'd always thought, well you know, she wasn't like the other girls, she was more, like, sensitive.

3: It is hereby agreed that at no time during the period of this contract shall The Datee draw attention to the following:

i: The Dater's choice of the second least expensive bottle of wine;

ii: The way The Dater tucks his napkin into his shirt collar;

iii: The Dater's belief that it is only a matter of time before Chris Rea makes it big again;

iv: That The Datee actually has no interest in whether Arsenal should have played Limpar, despite his injury, that afternoon, whatever Limpar is or, come to that, Arsenal.

4: In consideration for this and notwithstanding that everybody knows who Limpar is, small Swedish bloke, plays up front, The Dater undertakes:

i: Not to eat all the After Eights which come with the bill;

ii: Not to cause embarrassment to both parties by paying with any credit card that causes the waiter to ask The Dater whether he would mind stepping over to the till for just a second, thus making it clear to everybody in the restaurant that the Dater can't even run to a curry, let alone, and *inter alia*, a good bottle of wine.

5: At the termination of the meal The Dater agrees to conduct The Datee to her place of residence, always notwithstanding that should The Datee insist on travelling the seven miles home alone, on foot, through a derelict housing estate and a freight marshalling yard, The Dater shall take this as fair notice to quit.

6: Always provided that The Datee does not leave The Dater standing on the doorstep (ref: That Fool Nigel, passim) The Datee agrees the following:

  i: That she shall within 5 (five) minutes of crossing the threshold make it plain, by word or by deed, whether she is any of the following:

   a) Not That Sort of Girl.

   b) Not That Sort of Girl on a first date.

   c) Not That Sort of Girl after a dodgy curry and a warm bottle of Blue Nun.

   d) Entirely That Sort of Girl, but not with The Dater.

  ii: That at no point during the evening will The Datee introduce The Dater to her collection of soft toys which line her bed and get sulky if he refuses to greet each of them with the words 'How do you do, Teddy Nutkin?'

7: Should clauses 1 to 6 above be satisfied it is hereintofore agreed that neither party shall cause the following to be uttered:

  i: I don't do this with everyone I go out with, you know;

  ii: You will still respect me in the morning, won't you?;

  iii: I'd like to stay, honest, but I've got football training first thing. Now, where's my other sock?;

  iv: You won't tell anyone in the office about this, will you?;

  v: Damn! Look, er, I'm terribly sorry: this has never happened to me before;

  vi: Funny, that's not what Jennifer in Accounts Pending says.

The Times Magazine

FEBRUARY 1992

DOES MY BOTTOM LOOK TOO BIG?

SPEECHLESS IS NOT my usual state and, given an ear to bend, I am just the man to bend it until it hurts. But place me outside the changing room of a women's outfitters and ask me to comment on a newly outfitted woman and I am struck dumb. 'Yes,' I will say. 'It's sort of . . . yes. Isn't it?' It's not even as if I don't know about clothes. My grandfather ran a rather grand gents' suiting emporium in the West End of London, my mother spent my formative years designing whatever it was you and I were wearing through the Sixties and Seventies. Show me an A-line and I will tell you in which way it is not an Empire line; turn up your collar and I'll bore you with the details of the way in which the couturier has failed to set it properly into the body; let me mix it with the chaps who talk raglan sleeves and self-covered buttons and I am a man transported.

Until a woman comes out of the fitting room and says, 'You don't think it makes my bottom look too big, do you?' Do you *know* how impossible that question is to answer? Do you ever stop to think that there are men who have spent long years in the diplomatic corps pacifying belligerent dictators with the sweetest and most perfectly chosen phrases, who have stood in front of the stripped pine, mock saloon-bar changing rooms of some Champs-Elysées boutique or Fifth Avenue atelier quaking as they wait for their wives and mistresses to emerge with the absent-mindedly spoken but heart-stopping phrase, 'With my legs I probably need something longer, don't I?' I have met men who, with their honeyed oratory, can hold audiences in their hands at the National Theatre or at political party conferences but who, faced with a girlfriend trying on a new sweater at the local Top Shop, are struck dumb by the twelve sub-texts buried under the question, 'It's a really nice colour but doesn't it make me look flat-chested?'

The problem is that most women seem to view their bodies rather as a fly views a titbit left on the kitchen dresser. You will remember, I'm sure, doing the fly at school: that magnified eye with a thousand different facets, which gives it the ability to focus on minute specks of breadcrumb, and at the same time displays each crumb in a thousand different ways. So it is with the woman looking at her body.

At some very basic level she sees what the rest of the objective world sees: a naked body with its soft, rounded bits here and its hard, angular bits there, and its calloused bits where the pumice stone didn't work, and its bits that stand proud and its other bits which, gracefully or otherwise, have acknowledged the laws of gravity. She sees the textures, smooth and rough and crinkly and ridged and hairy, and she sees the colours where the veins come close to the skin or shy away from it, or where the sun has stayed too long or missed altogether or where the capillaries have broken and flooded the epidermis. She sees it as a surgeon may see it, or a camera. And she takes that vision and packs it away at the back of her mind where it may offer the least interference to the other visions – the visions which compare her to Linda Evangelista or the free 'n' easy type in the tampon add, or her husband's secretary or the girl next door. In *that* vision the wrinkles deepen into a geriatric's scar or disappear completely, the folds of flesh become voluptuous curves or corpulent great sacks of grease.

All of those visions are corrupted still further by the outside world. I have known women physicists who could write volumes on the reflection and refraction of light but still don't understand that looking down on their legs in a full-length mirror gives a foreshortened view of them, or that twisting their backs to see their bottoms in the same mirror shows only the hunched bottom of a person with a twisted back. Every friendly greeting of 'Lost weight?' takes a stone off, every pass by the optically unsound plate glass of a shop window puts two stone on.

And you're surprised that we all go silent on you when you ask whether the new mini makes your bum look fat? The problem is that while you're asking us for an aesthetic response (albeit one tempered by love or lust or our feeling for our secretary), what you are making yourself is a moral judgement. For shape and size isn't about what feels comfortable or even what looks good, but about what the fashion spread or the come-on ad says you *should* look like.

Hefty thighs – as they tell it – aren't an affront to art but to nature, and woman's natural estate is to be trim of ankle and narrow of beam with breasts like small and firm blancmanges. So what can we say when you ask whether the dress makes your legs look fat? We can always lie and say, 'No, darling – it makes them look slim and long,' but if you believed that you wouldn't have asked in the first place. Or we can say, 'Hey! Who cares, as long as I love you in it?' which is so entirely beside the point as to be fatuous. If your loved one's was the only view that mattered we would all walk around naked in the summer and wrapped in potato sacks in the winter. So we can tell a sort of truth and say, 'Well, it depends which way you stand. Perhaps if you wore it with those black stilettos at the bottom of the wardrobe . . .' Which can only translate as, 'Yes – your legs look fat, but on a different subject entirely, why don't you wear stilettos to bed any more?' Or we can tell the whole truth and say, 'Look, much as you want to be eighteen again with legs up to your armpits, you ain't. And, even if you were, then the pork pie and chips you had for lunch would make that dress an impossibility. And, even if it were a possibility, then you should know better by now than to try on a size 12 because the assistant says she hasn't got any 14s but that these ones are cut large. And that, even if you ignore all of that and still buy a dress two sizes too small for you, I'll be happy to be seen with you wearing it, because I love you and still retain the memory of what you looked like when you were size 10 with legs up to your armpits and all the way back down again. But would you mind not wearing it to the rugby club dinner-dance on Friday?'

The fact is that, 'What does this dress look like on me?' is unanswerable. There is no right answer because no woman can possibly conform to the dozen different varieties of perfection that are demanded of her. Or rather, that she demands of herself.

She

26 APRIL 1992

TRYING TIMES

GOD SAVE US all from the pub bore with his monogrammed pewter tankard and his lifetime of grievances; and God forgive the publisher who in some rash moment gives the pub bore a contract and an advance. Were it not for an unhappy confluence of time and place, His Honour Judge James Pickles (retd) would be sitting now by the fire in some mock-Tudor King's Arms or other, grabbing hapless strangers by the arm and telling them how, were it not for the old school ties, the cravenness of his erstwhile colleagues, the laziness of those who should know better and the treachery of womankind, he would, at the very least, be Lord Chief Justice.

James Pickles was a low-ranking judge on the north-western circuit, trying cases of robbery in Halifax and GBH in Bradford and occasionally writing an opinion piece for the papers, when his luck changed. A woman who was to appear as a prosecution witness against the boyfriend who had allegedly beaten her up, refused the stand: Pickles found her in contempt of court and gave her seven days. Another woman got pregnant in between her committal for theft and her appearance in court: Pickles gave her six months, saying that he didn't want to encourage others to believe that they could avoid jail by getting pregnant.

Both sentences excited the press, but then the press often gets excited by the eccentricities of our judges, most of whom believe that responding publicly to editorials shrieking 'Why this judge must go now!' is beneath their dignity. Not Pickles: after the second case made headlines, he called a full press conference in the three-ale bar of his local pub. Word soon got around Fleet Street that any journalist who needed a quote for a piece on the law need only give Pickles a ring. Jimmy Pickles, the Amazing Talking Judge, started taking his act around the heavyweight press, then the tabloids, got himself an agent, appeared three times on Wogan.

Ten years earlier, these antics would have had him out on his ear; as it was (Chapter 8, 'How Close Did I Come to Being Sacked?'), he started rattling his cage at around the same time that the constraints on judges were relaxed, and he managed to make it to retirement more or less unscathed. He hung up his wig last year and almost immediately took it off its peg again to serve as the stage prop he wears in his picture byline in the *Sun*.

The wisdom he has dispensed to the *Sun* and Terry Wogan, and that which he offered to Lord Hailsham (who never wrote back), is distilled in this tedious book and can be summed up in a few words: the judicial system is run by Oxbridge men who are more concerned with preserving the pomp of the courtroom than with dispensing justice; those in a position to do something about it won't because they are either scared of the Lord Chief Justice or on the lookout for a gong; solicitors are lazy moneygrabbers; judicial bureaucracy favours the lawyer rather than his client or the judicial system; female solicitors dress better than male ones; 'bobbling' women who don't wear bras should share the blame with any overwrought man who makes a lunge for their bosom; the police tend to stick together.

Pickles has a solution to these problems and the solution is that the Lord Chancellor or Lord Chief Justice should listen to Pickles. Indeed, some of Pickles's solutions have already been implemented, and while Pickles doesn't claim all the credit for himself he performs neat tricks by self-promotion: 'I have agitated for a fairer system of appointment, and there are recent signs that changes are being slowly made,' or, 'Lord Hailsham did, however, set up a Civil Justice Review body to examine court delays and related problems. I wondered whether my document had triggered this off . . .' Given that their relationship was roughly that which binds the chief rabbi to a ham sandwich, I doubt it.

The trouble is that much of the time and bobbling, bra-less women aside Pickles is absolutely right. More: when he has been wrong, he acknowledges the fact. He did perform some minor acts of judicial bravery, which may have changed the relationship between the press and the courts, and he has sacrificed any preferment he might have achieved by speaking his mind. But his leaden prose style and his pusillanimous temperament turn the common-sense thought and the reasoned argument into a boastful, recreant tirade.

After a couple of chapters minutely detailing how he refused costs to solicitors who wasted the court's (i.e. Pickles's) time, or his mealy-mouthed praise of his seniors ('Lord Justice Harry Woolf is very clever; I have only met him once, briefly, but have heard nothing to his disadvantage') or of his sudden plummets into *Sun*-speak ('Come off it, Scrivener!') I began to believe that those superannuated ogres of the judiciary who snubbed Pickles can't, by that simple definition, be all bad.

Sunday Times

Review of *Judge for Yourself* by His Honour Judge Pickles (Smith Gryphon, 1992)

8 OCTOBER 1992

WHEN A FILM SCRIPT BECOMES

REAL LIFE

THERE YOU ARE sitting in the pub and somebody says did you see this stuff about Michael Douglas booking in to a clinic to get his sex addiction sorted, somebody else says, hey, me and Michael both, difference is I can't get a sick note from the doctor for it, and there you are wondering bemusedly whether a) there is any such thing as sex addiction, b) whether you're addicted too, and c) if you are whether you can claim it as an excuse the next time you get caught *in flagrante* with Helga the au pair. (I had thought, progressive 1990s man that I am, to run that as a unisexual lure addressed to women as well as men. But who are we kidding here?)

I understand your confusion and I am here to set your mind at rest.

Let us first dispense with the case of Michael Douglas. Douglas is a very rich, very powerful man working in Hollywood. Fifteen times a day he will be approached by 19-year-old women of astonishing beauty and incredibly short skirts, who will ask him for sex. Sex in Rodeo Drive restaurants, sex across the desks of film studio offices, sex in the Paramount Pictures broom cupboard. Once, sometimes twice, a week a producer will phone him up and say 'Hey! Mikey! Baby! Boychik! I got this script it's absolutely built for you Mikey.' And Douglas says, 'Does it involve doing it in a broom cupboard with three 19-year-old women in incredibly short skirts?' And the producer says, 'How come you know the plot already? That schmendrick writer, he promised me nobody else even seen this script.'

I will grant, given the above, that Michael Douglas might have the odd problem relating to women and that his life's creed might indeed start with the words 'If it moves . . .'. But this is no help for the rest of us. What the rest of us want to know is, are we as other men, if not better? That is all men really want to know. When we find ourselves changing seats on the train the better to make eye or leg contact with the woman who we would swear has been taking sly glimpses in our direction, is that sex addiction? When we turn a lunch date into a dinner date on some feeble pretext, or we try to persuade our wives and girlfriends to wear something more revealing and less suitable, is that sex addiction?

I'm no expert, but I doubt it. Were thought not only mother to the deed but its identical twin sister as well then every window-shopper would be arrested for shoplifting. The Pope, according to one of his more memorably unworldly encyclicals, might not be able to distinguish the thought of adultery from the deed but, as is so often the case with his Holiness, that's easy for him to say, isn't it?

The reason I'm so loath to believe in sexual addiction is that I can only really think of addictions as those habits which are available to us all. Anybody can become a kleptomaniac; alcoholism is no respecter of class or bank balance as any once-comfortably off meths drinker will tell you. But sex addiction is only available to those of us who have access to a supply of the addictive material. And most men haven't.

I assume, by the way, that sex addiction is a defence only open to those men who are in some sort of steady relationship. I'd guess that were I a New York therapist searching for a new field of practice I'd be able to persuade a few men who, unattached, are happy sleeping in a different bed every night that their lifestyle was dangerously psychopathic. The fact is, though, that most of the men who live that way enjoy themselves no end, and however much you tell them about the love of a good woman and the usefulness of knowing that when you wake up in the morning the post on the doormat is yours, they can't see what the problem is.

But when I think of all the married and long-term partnered men I know I can think of perhaps one or two for whom sex addiction is any sort of option at all. Their partners may have grown to love their paunches and their thinning hair, their habit of turning every conversation round to QPR's chances in the Cup, their quirks of personal hygiene, but the rest of the world, and especially that female and available section of it, finds all that an unacquirable taste. True: these men may have the occasional affair and if the partnership broke up they may eventually find another partner, but sex is not an addiction open to them.

I can't believe, though, that none of these men has a sex drive as powerful as Michael Douglas's, or that if they had whatever it is that Douglas has they wouldn't use it in the way that he has apparently been using it. Let us assume, then, that there are thousands of men around who, were they Douglas, would be doing what he does. They aren't so they can't. What Douglas has can't, therefore, be an addiction. QE, I rather think, D.

What we have in Douglas, then, is not a sex addict but an old-fashioned philanderer. And in Diandra, who sent him for therapy, we have not an addict's wife, but somebody who copes with her husband's philandering by giving it a fancy name which suggests that he is somehow more virile, more desirable than other husbands on her street. He may be, but addiction has nothing to do with it.

The Times Magazine

124

12 MAY 1994

CALL ME PICKY

NEVER MIND THE Gault-Millau stars and the English Tourist Board crowns and the Michelin castles: there are only three types of hotel in Britain. If we're spending somebody else's money we stay in hotels where the chambermaid folds the loose end of the lavatory paper into a neat triangle each day, and if we're spending our own money we stay in hotels where she leaves the loose end of the paper hanging free. Under all circumstances we try to avoid the third type, the lavatory paper of which you are currently reading because all they've left you is a cardboard tube with a single sheet on it.

Believe me, I know: I've just spent a week on the road staying in the best provincial hotels Britain has to offer and the good news is that when you ask for a junior suite in the excellent Crowne Plaza in Manchester they give you one of that town's smaller boroughs to sleep in. The bad news is that I only felt justified in asking for a junior suite because of where I'd stayed the night before and where I was pretty certain I'd have to stay the night after.

I offer you, for instance, the hotel in Chesterfield which is part of a chain which incorporates an Edinburgh hotel, where the receptionist once told me brightly that she didn't put through my ordered alarm call because she thought I was probably sleeping. The Chesterfield outpost of this happy chain is stuck tantalisingly on the unreachable side of a road which is cut off by works on the town's sewage system. I spent an extra £4 to get myself an 'executive room' and, although I've never executed a thing in my life, I've met real executives and I know that they're not accustomed to their bedcovers having been used to help mop up the mess caused by works being carried out on the town's sewers down the road. Fair enough: that's an exaggeration. I'm prepared to believe that the cover had just borne the weight of three of the town's more popular hookers for a couple of sessions while they tried to keep their feet off the sticky carpet.

Whatever: the room at least had a mini-bar, which, I happen to know, is the only thing executives look for in a hotel room once they've discovered that the television doesn't show dirty movies. The mini-bar contained just the one item: a sheet of rumpled paper which told me that if I fancied a drink there were some miniatures stored behind the reception desk.

It wasn't just Chesterfield, though. In every one of the Midlands towns I went through I had the choice of a fusty B&B, a newly thrown up set of fifty-quid-a-night barracks next to Toys "Я" Us on the ring road or another decrepit and sticky-carpeted railway hotel. And anyone anticipating buying shares in InterCity who thinks that any enterprise passed from BR ownership to that of the private sector automatically becomes a haven of bright efficiency should try staying at one of the northern ex-railway hotels. Call me picky, but it's not good enough. In the US, every one-horse town has its own spruce Sheraton competing with its own jaunty Marriott, and either will give me a clean room with a mini-bar and all the dirty movies I need for the same price as the English road-ring barracks. America, I know, is different: the porter in the Marriott is more biddable than his English counterpart because he believes that one day he will own the hotel. The poor sap won't, of course, but it doesn't stop him believing. And American towns are further from other American towns than are English towns from each other, which means that while I can get to Leeds and back in a day without having to stop over, the chances are that a trip from anywhere to Spittoon will mean a night in the Spittoon Hotel.

That only explains why they have more hotels, though; it does nothing to explain why our small-town hotels are so awful.

If Chesterfield has a market for hotel rooms at all then it

must surely have one for rooms with clean bedcovers and a mini-bar policy which doesn't assume you're Olly Reed set on a heavy night. How much more can it cost to build and run a hotel that people want to stay in rather than one which they are prepared to stay in if pushed?

What is most depressing of all is that the hotel guides and the star-awarding tourist boards conspire in all this mediocrity. The Chesterfield establishment got its stars, I guess, because any hotel with a carpet automatically gets a couple of points in order to teach carpetless hotels a lesson or because some middle manager decided that putting gold-tapped bidets in the executive rooms is a reasonable trade-off against keeping the bedcovers in use for a couple of extra years. It isn't, and the next time I see an American bellboy who reckons that one day he'll own his own hotel, I'll send him to the Chesterfield, where there is a small fortune to be made.

The Times Magazine

18 JUNE 1994

BABY BORE

IT JUST GOES to show, eh? You think you know who your friends are, and then this.

A woman sends *The Times Magazine* a letter (4 June) complaining about my child, my daughter, my little defenceless baby, who has done nobody any harm, a woman who goes by the name of Helen Gobat – and they publish it. Like they haven't got enough letters, right? Like there aren't thousands of reasonable, well-balanced *Times* readers out there complaining about the excess of stick-thin totty on the fashion pages, or about Anne Robinson's hair, or the Meades stomach; like they couldn't have slipped the letter into the bin, and who would have known? But no.

What this Gobat woman says – and it's not like she's going to have to fork out for the therapy in twenty years when the arm's-length object of her derision comes across the letter in some dusty cuttings file – is that I've become a baby bore.

Damn right I have. And she doesn't know the half of it. In a week I have done the following:

Fixed three men, variously eight, ten and eighteen years younger than me, with my most serious eye and told them that they really ought to start a family now because they don't want to leave it as late as I did.

Heard myself saying, brightly, 'Well, I suppose it'll be you two next,' to assorted childless couples who are happy with their estate.

Had lunch with a wildly attractive and unattached twenty-two-year-old woman and, over the soup course, showed her

128

the three pictures of my baby which I keep in my wallet.

Drunk water while lunching said twenty-two-year-old.

Asked a friend if he wouldn't mind smoking out in the garden.

Bought a roof rack.

Bought one of those things for holding cans of drink steady on long car journeys.

When asked what size nicotine chewing gum I wanted at the chemists, found myself answering, 'Oh you know: the family size.'

Thought about going to Ikea.

Booked a holiday without telling a travel editor.

Discovered myself to have an opinion on the hydroscopic capabilities of Pampers.

Bought a house because of its garden and its proximity to a reputable junior school, regardless of its being further away from the club I drink at.

Not drunk at my club for a month.

Heard myself complaining about violence on television.

Found myself reading Bernard Levin's column and nodding meaningfully at it.

Picked up my saxophone and opened *Classic R&B Hits of the Sixties*, only to find myself trying to work out an obbligato for 'Horsey Horsey Don't You Stop'.

Heard myself barking to a couple having a loudish conversation in the next-door garden at 7pm, 'Do you mind? There's a baby trying to sleep!'

Engaged a senior nurse in a heated argument about breast-feeding.

Found myself starting arguments with, 'Yes, I suppose that's all very well in theory, but just you wait until you've got kids . . .'

Driven very slowly and stopped for people who might possibly be walking in the general direction of the zebra crossing, but who are still sixty yards away.

Phoned my parents three times in a week.

Started reading the nutritional-value information on the back of rusk packets.

Told a woman queuing in front of me at the Sainsbury's

checkout that, actually, those baby-wipes can leave a bit of a nasty rash.

Smiled at policemen.

Spent two hours trying to find old editions of *The Family from One End Street* and *Milly-Molly-Mandy*.

Started at least three sentences with 'You know, much as I love London . . .'

As a result, Ms Gobat, you'll be pleased to know that, in a fit of anxiety, I sold my child to a passing Romanian couple who took a fancy to her. She is, I understand, making a sort of life for herself in Bucharest. I, meanwhile, have taken to riding fast motorbikes again, smoking heavily and flirting dangerously with Take That fans. I can only hope you're very pleased with yourself.

The Times Magazine

24 September 1994

SOGGY BREAD EXISTS IN
THREE DIMENSIONS

FOR THE PAST nine months I have watched her studying the unstudiable, repeating the most banal motions, making chaos I never realised was possible out of an order I never knew was there. The baby books, in their facile way, tell me this is part of the learning process. I know better:

Abstracts from the Proceedings of the Royal Institute of Everything
　　President: Cosima Lawson-Diamond FRIE

1 Department of Physics
A certain piece of bread of consistent weight n was repeatedly allowed to fall from a walking frame q. In between each event the bread was soaked in saliva for a period lasting no longer than p seconds, where p equals the maximum time the experimenter's attention can be sustained by the stain on the floor. Demonstrated: that soggy bread exists in three dimensions, viz: space, time and carpet.

2 Department of Applied Psychology
An experimental subject, J, was invited to place a pair of expensive spectacles on his nose, which were repeatedly removed by the experimental staff and allowed to fall to the floor. Each time, the experimenter noted carefully the subject's subsequent action. The experimenter also giggled a lot. In some 98 per cent of cases – based on a sample of 563 – the subject replaced the spectacles on his nose, disproving all past

behavioural studies regarding the learning abilities of the major primates. Demonstrated: that the behaviour of rats in previous laboratory experiments bears no obvious relation to that of humans, given that rats would have switched to contact lenses after the first half-dozen experiments.

3 Department of Environmental Science

Our experimenters attempted to demonstrate that it was possible to conserve many of the world's diminishing softwood forests by stretching the products of their trees to fill a greater area. Using the formula $z=cx^3$, where z equals the size in square metres of a surface and c represents the extent to which any given newspaper is as yet unread, it was demonstrated that in the time (p) it takes to put a bowl of junior pasta in the microwave, the *Ealing Gazette* can be shredded in such a way as to cover an average sitting-room carpet to a depth of x.

4 Department of Materials Science

One group of assistants was sent to buy a number of extremely expensive items of laboratory equipment from the latest Early Learning Centre and leave them in the laboratory next to the nappy basin. A second group was asked to leave apparently worthless items – bits of old shoelace, twigs, spent matches, keys from sardine cans – hidden about the laboratory. After some weeks of experimentation it was determined that the ratio of scientific interest in any given item to its cost is expressed by the formula $E/(3-xp\ (h))$, where E is the time, in nanoseconds, it takes to drop a Bibblee Bobblee Play'n'Learn Activity Table and h is the time in hours it is possible to play with a piece of dry and fluffy toast found behind the sofa.

5 Department of Human Anatomy

Having done much research on the major extremities and discovered that under all experimental conditions – beneath blanket, behind cot, in bath water, with bath water all over bathroom floor – there remain two hands and two feet, we attempted to demonstrate that the inside of a subject's lower lip remained constantly bruised when scraped with a fingernail ten times a day.

6 Department of Parapsychology

We have endeavoured to demonstrate how an experimenter who is less than three feet tall and unable yet to walk properly may, through power of thought alone, cause a four-foot-high shelf of books to manifest itself on the floor. Further papers from the Department of Food Ballistics, the Biting Research Working Party and the Rusk Adhesion Panel will appear in future editions of the Proceedings.

The Times Magazine

3 December 1994

ANIMISM

ANIMISM HAS SERVED the Burmese pretty well these past few hundred years. Persuade the man on the bus to Mandalay that his rubber tree and his three-piece suite share the same spirit and he'll live happily without irritable bowel syndrome or repetitive strain injury or ME or any of the ills with which we non-animists are burdened and which the Burmese manage without.

Which is, I guess, why Britain is turning all animist and why it is only a matter of months before your children will be asked by their headmaster each morning to close their eyes and put their hands together and say thank you to the school cat for letting them get all the way to school without having their dinner money thumped out of them by the malign spirit living behind the bus shelter.

You will have noticed a lot of fuss recently about herbs and the people who prescribe herbs with rather more vim than my doctor prescribes Valium. The suits in Brussels have ordained that such prescription should be controlled by 117 separate Eurodirectives and that herbalists swap their bunches of dusty twigs and shredded leaves for neat little boxes with Essence of Shredded Leaf BP printed on the side in six languages. In retaliation the herbalists have shaven their beards, swapped their sandals for neat Clarks lace-ups, and mounted a campaign of reprisal.

For the most part this means sharing a cup of camomile tea with the more impressionable sort of mid-market women's editor and telling her about the wonder that is mother nature's private dispensary and the naked evil that is Dr Patel's Saturday Morning Surgery. This is the sort of thing which, according to one such women's editor, the herbalists are saying:

'Chemical drugs generally have a specific agenda, while herbs, through a complex biochemical process, take the whole person into consideration and replenish the body on a cellular level.'

Tell me: is this animism or is this animism?

You and I know and the herbalist knows that the world isn't split into chemicals and non-chemicals. Everything is chemicals: the Prozac tablet and the aspirin and the powdered willow bark and the shredded feverfew. Indeed, the only difference between the willow bark and the aspirin is that I can be pretty sure that one of them is as pure as Bayer can make it and isn't mixed in with the slimier bits of whatever was crawling over the other one before it was felled to make a dozen cricket bats and a handful of mother nature's headache remedy.

Give a moderately adept chemist any herbal remedy and he'll give you back a list of all the chemicals in it, and no garbage about which particular agent is the kindly animist one which takes the whole person into consideration. He could doubtless perform the same trick on the 'natural ecstasy' which was reported the other week as being imported, quite legally, from Australia. That nobody has yet analysed the natural drug seems, as far as I can see, only to encourage the naturopaths: the less we know about it the more wonderfully natural it remains, and never mind that you hit the pavement with the same dull thud when you try to fly on the natural brand.

But wait: we have proof here. According to our herbalist, the Princess of Wales started on homeopathic remedies and then moved on to aromatherapy, acupuncture, colonic irrigation, osteopathy and reflexology. What an advert that is, eh? Nothing there about the natural fingers going down the natural throat after every natural fish supper. Or what about Axl Rose, the noted homeopathic patient who 'flew into a rage when security men ordered him to hand over his medicine to be X-rayed'. So much for natural remedies – and I quote our herbalist again – 'not upsetting the body's natural harmony'.

In fact as far as I can see everyone who is ever trotted out as an example of what natural medicine can do has rather more ailments, real or imagined, than those who survive on aspirin and Andrews Liver Salts. Indeed, the function of all natural medicines seems not to be to cure you but to let you be at one with your neuroses.

All of which is just fine by me. Pile high the shelves of Boots with every mud-caked weed you can find, and man the barricades when the Brussels suits try to stop you. But don't pretend that the weeds or, come to that, the mud, aren't as much chemical compositions as the little white pills they replace. Because if they have something other than chemicals then it would have to be something that only the Burmese animist could describe.

The Times Magazine

7 JANUARY 1995

COLUMN GONE

Sit down at desk, switch on computer, look for half-written column. Good column, all about letter from insurance company offering free travel alarm clock if give them pleasure of betting against me falling off perch and how come insurance companies think Taiwanese travel alarm clock suitable inducement to make major financial decision. Three medium-good gags, two gobbets genuine wisdom, still only halfway through. Column gone. Odd.

Look through folders to find 'documents' folder in which stored column.

Whole bloody 'documents' folder gone. Weird.

Now short by one half-written column, one article for women's magazine, letter to agent, ditto to VAT man, sundry other things which won't know about until angry editors start phoning asking where hell is copy, deadline week ago, what hell think playing at, call self professional?

Do not panic.

Have been writing by computer since 1983: have yet to lose single piece of copy. Am expert on recovering copy from dusty trouser turn-ups of hard disk. People phone up, say, 'John – copy gone. Help!', pop round, press buttons, magic! Copy reappears, accept large drink, promise of meal, money, use of wife.

Deep breath.

Open special copy-recovery program. Have large drink while program looks behind virtual sofa, under virtual rug, down back of virtual lavatory cistern for lost copy. OK: two large drinks given that already have use of own wife.

Back at desk. List on screen of 927 items of copy previously disposed of. What insurance piece called? Insurance? 'Cannot find file "Insurance"' appears on screen. Alarm clock? 'Cannot find file "Alarm Clock".' Open recovered files at random: like looking through virtual loft. 'Memo. From: John Diamond; To: Robert Maxwell . . . 047'; 'Dear Sir, re your ad in today's *UK Press Gazette* for a motorbike journalist . . . 047'; 'Jenny, about your not showing up on Friday . . .' Magic moments.

Hour later. Large drink. Wife gone out. Door slammed. Sue Apple computers temporary loss of use of wife, half bottle whisky.

Screen full of recovered copy. Recovered copy impenetrable: recovery program recovers copy complete with every letter ever mistyped and corrected, every second, third, fourth thought. 'The quoickest way easiest way to get San Hose Jose to is on by with BritisDelta Airwaysline & but . . .' Some copy imponderably wiser than ever knew: 'with life like lifelike basin off cool darkness'. Even deconstructed what could ever have meant? Whyever have written it?

Sudden flash of computer-guru inspiration. Still not panicking. Have large drink. What was inspirational flash again? Flash comes back: try to recreate documents folder. Open general controls; click on 'Create documents folder'. If documents folder created then surely contents – half-written column, piece for women's mag, VAT letter etc – will appear with it. Computer goes 'boing'; being computer guru have set computer to go boing instead of beep. Thought it v. witty until about five seconds ago.

Message flashes on screen: 'Unable to create documents folder – Error – 127'. Click on little computer guru program to tell me what hell Error – 127 means. Error – 127 means Internal File System Error. What hell Internal File System Error?

Switch computer off, switch on again. Still not there. New inspirational flash – perhaps on wife's computer after all. Switch on wife's computer. Wife's computer go beep, lights go out. Mend fuse. Switch on own computer, start to write column from scratch.

'The other day I received a letter from an insurance company . . . 047.'

What was gag? Had gag there am sure. In brackets between 'letter' and 'from'. Good gag. What gag possibly fit there? No such gag. Must find gag. Gag not used is gag wasted. Might never be writing about insurance again, gag sitting there, impotent, in ether. Start second recovery program. Screen seizes up mid-boing. Restart computer: change boing to beep. Computer freezes again. Restart: little smiley computer appears on screen. Nothing else appears on screen. Move to hit smug git smiley computer on screen with whisky bottle, draw back at last moment, whisky pours over pile of disks.

Take deep breath. Count to ten. Logical order: reload system file, restart computer, write gentle piece – no gags – on travelling alarm clocks from scratch. Find system disk: system disk drenched in whisky. Lick whisky off disk. Put disk in computer. Computer rejects disk. Shut down computer. Go downstairs to use wife's computer. Wife back, using own computer. Wife says, 'Finished column? Where whisky?'

Sit at desk. Hit computer. Hit empty whisky bottle. Cry.

I got a letter in the post from an insurance company . . .

The Times Magazine

18 March 1995

TWENTY WAYS TO TELL YOU'RE

MIDDLE-AGED

FRIDAY NIGHT, LAST week. It is getting on for midnight in the middle of London, the pubs have chucked out and I'm standing on the pavement with some people I work with a couple of days each week. They are young people, people in their twenties, people who have to screw up their smooth faces and think hard to work out my too-frequent references to the Wilson years or Norman Vaughan. We are all after-work drunk and going on to a party.

I close my eyes and hear the familiar sounds: the cheap, party-booze bottles clinking in the thin plastic bags, the over-bright giggling, the benign but neighbour-waking bellows of a tipsy gang who can't begin to understand why the neighbours might be asleep before midnight on a Friday night when there's such a good time to be had here on the pavement.

They are, I realise, the Friday-midnight sounds of my youth. Their youth, too, I guess. It's just that we have different youths.

I go home and leave them to their party. No, it's not that I'm too old for this, I tell them: it's just that it's been a long day and I just want to be in bed, my bed, asleep.

I feel, although I am not, middle-aged. Rather, it is as if I am still a young man allowed a sudden miserable revelation that I don't have to stay out late on Fridays or go out at all on Saturday night to know I'm living a life.

Then again, middle age, said Ogden Nash rather too pointedly for my liking, is hearing the phone ring on while you're sitting at home on Saturday night and hoping it isn't for you.

Perhaps Nash was right. I'm forty-one, and if I'm not middle-aged then who is?

A couple of years ago my kid brother – at thirty-five he's still my kid brother – had some old super-8 holiday film transferred on to a video. The film was almost as old as my brother: he's there toddling about a drizzly Westcliff or Margate, my other brother is making faces into the lens and I'm a seven- or eight-year-old, jerkily spading damp sand, licking 99 cones, kicking a beachball in that ungainly way children have.

Overseeing the three of us is a smiling middle-aged man. Middle-aged haircut, middle-aged sweater, middle-aged shoes. A man who knows his responsibilities, who knows he has nothing to do with the teenagers and the twenty-year-olds hanging around on the beach. It isn't until the end of the film that it comes to me that the middle-aged man in the film, my father then in his mid-thirties, is younger then than I was as I watched him.

So why was he middle-aged and, glib old Ogden Nash notwithstanding, I'm not?

It's not just that he had three children by the age of thirty-five and I've just had my first. Nor can I quite convince myself that it's all a matter of attitude, despite what I find in those books of wacky quotations listing wry definitions of middle age from Bennett Cerf and Bob Hope and, of course, Ogden Nash. Yes, of course, I know people who bought their first grey Marks & Spencer suit at twenty and, more worrying still, used a Marks' charge-card to pay for it, and others who affect a perky and tedious youthfulness as they pick up their pension giro, but those people seem to exist outside the definitions. Or they would if there were any definitions left to exist outside, because there is no official definition of middle age.

Old age and youth are easily defined: at eighteen you're an adult, at sixty-five pensionable, at seventy-five you'll automatically be carted off to the geriatric wing if something goes wrong with you. But no insurance company, nor any employment agency, could tell me what middle age is. I could hear the shrug of their shoulders over the phone, and their invariable answer, translated, was always the same: middle age is what happens to other people.

Pushed, Britain's biggest insurance company, the Prudential, refused to acknowledge the concept: 'We don't use it in our literature any more,' a spokeswoman said. 'We use the term mid-life.'

This sounds more mathematical than anything else, but the way the Pru uses the term assumes an average age in three figures: mid-life for them starts at forty-five and lasts for another twenty years.

Mathematically, I suppose, middle age is thirty-six for men and thirty-eight for women, but that would make Keith Chegwin and Jonathan Ross middle-aged, which can't be right. The dictionary defines the term as 'the period between youth and old age' and says it has been in use since the seventeenth century, a period when the average lifespan was in the high forties and the mathematical middle age that of most of those who left me last Friday to go to the party.

The nearest I can get to a useful definition is a medical one from Archie Young, Professor of Geriatric Medicine at the Royal Free Hospital in north London. To be honest, Professor Young says, the rot for most things has already set in for me. 'Things like muscle strength are decreasing by the mid-40s. Or that's the average, at least: it covers a range from 25 to 55.' My muscles might have been winding down for fifteen years already, then.

We talk about some more organs. Why, for instance, and to pluck a phenomenon entirely at random, has my hangover changed in the past five years? Once I could have a few drinks from time to time and know that the worst that would happen would be a thick head when I woke up. Now I wake feeling sort of OK, and then, at around midday, feel I'm about to die and because the wakeful gap between drinking and hangover is so long I don't associate one with the other and really think I am going to die.

But perhaps middle age is knowing that dying is always a chance.

Professor Young tells me that my kidneys and my liver are probably getting weaker, and that my muscles are too, and we agree that, medically at least, I'm middle-aged. But then, what do doctors know? It is a commonplace belief that man is at his sexual peak at eighteen, so, if the state is defined by the first instance of decrepitude, it would make any randy nineteen-year-old ready for the comfy slippers and the pension plan.

Certainly when my father was being fatherly on the beach he looked like a man who knew he was middle-aged: looking back at the movie, even he sees a middle-aged man there. He's revised his definitions, though in a way which makes them even more slippery than my own defensive position on the matter, for although he agrees that the man in the film looks middle-aged, he says that he didn't begin to feel middle-aged until he was in his mid-fifties and his sons started getting married. My father isn't unique, though: something has happened to allow all of us to shift around our age groups, to slip into middle age and then slip out of it again for a while.

Perhaps it's that the hierarchy of age has changed.

Once maturity, seriousness, the straight-faced gravitas of middle age, was something to be striven for. Youth and young adulthood was a period of effective disenfranchisement, a time of apprenticeship and indentureship to those who had the knowledge, the power, the responsibility. It made sense for any twenty-five-year-old to want to behave like the forty-five-year-old, to dress like him, to speak like him, to swap the Woodbines for a pipe. Middle age, then, came at the period when the imitation of middle age started to look convincing at around thirty-five or so.

But I was born into an age when youth culture was everything, when only the youthful got whatever was worth having. It was the young who had the money, the laughs, the power. The corollary was that thirty or thirty-five or forty was death. And when we got to those ages and found that we didn't die after all. We just worried about dying.

But there were other changes as well. Twenty years ago the generational strata kept to themselves. When I was twenty the only people I knew were twenty and neither sixteen-year-olds nor twenty-five-year-olds came to my parties, nor I to theirs. But at the last party I threw there were a couple of eighteen-year-olds at one end of the range and a few sixty-year-olds at the other, and neither seemed to think it odd that they or the others were there.

Perhaps that's because some of the other generational definers have gone.

First it was clothes. When my parents were growing up there was no such thing as teenage clothes or styles peculiar to the young: there were children's clothes and grown-up clothes, and those who wore the latter had, sartorially at least, already started drifting towards middle age.

The teddy boys brought with them the idea of a uniform strictly for the young and the various groups of the 1960s – mods, rockers, skinheads, hippies – expanded on it. But then it all started getting a little confusing. Certainly when I was wearing loon pants and tie-dye T-shirts there were few men of my current age aping me, because forty-year-olds still wore a white shirt and a dark suit to work. Now, though, most of those divisions are gone. True, I would have looked pretty stupid in the purposeful raggedness of grunge rather than the accidental raggedness I usually affect, and I couldn't quite bring myself to dress in flares when they made a brief reappearance a couple of years ago. On the other hand, I buy most of my clothes sharing a communal changing-room with men twenty years younger or older than me. Stranger still is that while I'll often wear a suit and tie out of preference, my father, a man whose first pink shirt I can still remember, is invariably kitted out in the leisure-jacket style that is the hallmark of the modern pensioner.

It's not true that there are no sartorial boundaries to distinguish the young from the old, but they have become as fuzzy as any other distinction between the two groups seems to be.

Or take music. The music I listened to as a teenager was almost nothing like that which my parents liked: everything changed in the 1950s and then again in the 1960s. They had be bop and big bands, I had the Beatles. But while the musical continuum was interrupted every decade or so for the first half of the century, since I started buying Golden Guinea albums popular music has stayed much the same.

True, there have been punk and hip hop and a dozen other genres which I happily slept through and affect not to understand, as if three guys beating the hell out of a synthesiser takes any understanding, but rather more connects the culture of Whigfield with that of the Dave Clark Five than holds together Dave Clark and Mario Lanza.

The stock-holding, country-house dwelling quinquagenarians of the 1960s and 1970s rock are still doing as good business now as they were then, and not merely among those who have grown up with them. Is Jagger middle-aged? Or Clapton? Or McCartney? Well, yes, McCartney's always been middle-aged, but, if Lennon were still with us, would he be?

Yes, of course, but only because if we have to have a middle age then being fifty must be it, regardless of how loud you like to play your music.

The truth is that the divisions between ages have gone the way of the divisions between classes. Once there were three easily distinguishable classes and you could place a man in one or another by his job, his aspirations, his clothes, his accent. Now there is a large, but by no means dominant, underclass, a working-class rump, and everyone else has a job and a roof over their head and is, by the new definition, middle class.

Just as the ABC1 class definitions of the economists tell only half the social story, so the chronological ages of the population describe only one small aspect of what we are. There are the obviously young and the undeniably old, and everyone else is whatever they want to be. Sure, rich and tubby old geezers in baggy rock-star suits escorting women whose legginess has nothing to do with support tights are still faintly ridiculous, but no more so than rich and tubby young geezers who use their money to play the same trick. Age has stopped being a determining factor in these things.

The editors of all our broadsheet daily and Sunday papers, for instance, are in their forties, and some of them only just. The editor of the *Sunday Telegraph* is still in his thirties, albeit going on fifty, and the boy at the *News of the World*, the biggest-selling paper of them all, is in his twenties, damn him.

Once newspaper proprietors wouldn't consider granting an editorship to anyone who hadn't reached positive middle age, but since middle age has become indefinable, that hardly works any more.

It's not that there's no such thing as middle age: by any definition I am of, or about to be of, it. What distinguishes my middle age from my father's is that I am of a group which, in the 1960s, dispensed with the old bias against the young. We are the ones who grew up proud of our youth rather than ashamed of it and, as we've got older, we've simply moved our pride up a notch. We got to being the right age, the correct age, the age which had everything going for it. Why should we give all that up?

And so we have baggaged up our music and our clothes and our whole having-it-all inheritance, and we have translated it for a new age. Our market-stall design style has become Habitat, our Oxfam clothes come from Paul Smith or Next. We were once young and felt pity for those who weren't; now we are middle-aged and feel the same patronising pity for the young.

We are, as we always have been, and as we used to say when I was young, where it's at.

The Times Magazine

15 April 1995

HE'S ME

YOU KNOW THE bloke standing at the front of the queue in the post office waving a crumpled piece of paper?

The one complaining that it never used to be like this and that he can remember a day when if you posted a letter with the name on it but, for some bizarre reason which seems to have slipped his mind pro tem, no address, the post office – the old post office that is, the one staffed by forensic postmen wise to the ways of the absent-minded, men who could divine a missing address from the merest hint of soup stain on the envelope – would deliver it, unlike your modern post office which took three days to get this very important Reader's Digest You May Already Have Won a Rover 280 offer back whence it came, and can he speak to a supervisor, please: no, not when he's finished counting the bloody postal orders, but now. You know him?

He's me.

He never used to be me. Once I was you, squirming with embarrassment and impatience halfway along the queue, but now I'm that bloke, and I can't say I like him much.

True, I was never one quietly to let a waiter pass a cold steak off as a hot supper and I've been known to raise an eyebrow at any barman who serves three inches of froth, but this Colonel Blimp routine is all new to me, like waking up one morning and finding all you've got in the wardrobe are cavalry twills and small-check Viyella shirts.

For instance: I have this routine I do with London cabs. The Public Carriage Office says they have to follow strict rules, like taking me back to Shepherd's Bush when they really want to go to the Savoy so they can tell Americans that the big orange one with the silver stripe is really a tenner.

When they don't follow the rules I make this big deal about noting down their number as they're driving away. I never do anything with the number – indeed a couple of times when I've not been able to find a pen I've mimed the whole thing with the blunt end of my finger – but if they can give me a moment of irritation by not taking my fare, I can return the favour by pretending I'm going to report them.

Except the other week I did it. I wanted to go west to work, he wanted to go east and home, I said but hold on, your light's up, he said . . . whatever. And for the first time I sat down and wrote a letter to the Public Carriage Office, which office has just written back to me to say the cabby has had his wrist slapped.

Do I feel better for hearing the slap? Do I feel better for shouting at the bin men when they leave a curl of potato peel at my gate, or at the manager at Texas Homecare when I find for the third visit running they had part (a) but had run out of part (b) which gives part (a) its reason for being – in the latest case a rack full of broom heads but no broom handles?

When did I stop being the sort of man who picks up the potato peel and puts it in the empty dustbin or the sort who shrugs and goes to B&Q for his broom? When did I develop the haughty voice you need to say things like, 'Excuse me, but I think you've dropped something' to small boys who toss their lolly wrappers into the gutter, and 'I think you'll find I was here first' to queue-jumpers?

A new honesty? Not really: I've always been irritated by cabbies and handle-less brooms, it's just that until recently I was quietly irritated. A sense of public service? Obviously not, given the muttering noise the queuing public makes behind me. The ageing process? Well, perhaps. Maybe we all have special crustiness genes programmed to trip into action when we hit a certain age, members of the same gene species which set us writing letters to the local paper and joining committees and wearing cavalry twill.

But yesterday I found myself behind a querulous old git at

Sainsbury's and, as he argued the toss with the blameless cashier about the price of yoghurt, I discovered my old self again. I wanted to tell him to shut up and let the rest of us get on with our shopping. Instead, I squirmed cravenly and waited my turn and heard myself saying to the cashier, 'You'd think they'd have better things to get upset about, wouldn't you?'

The Times Magazine

19 AUGUST 1995

THE UNIFIED THEORY OF

HORTICULTURAL SCIENCE

OH, BUT THE novel I shall write, the concerto I'll compose, the home I shall build, and just as soon as I discover the one tiny thing which is standing in my way. For there is always just the one thing, and it is always so tiny.

Each day this summer, for instance, I have gone out of the back door and I have looked at the yellow and matted lawn and the limp, bone-coloured daisies melding into the dust-bowl which is the herbaceous border, and the peach-leaf curl which has, against all the tenets of gardening wisdom, become peach-twig curl and has started to become unidentified-shrub-next-to-peach-tree curl too. And at the wormy apples lying in squishy brown heaps at the base of an apple tree. And I have understood that if I knew the one thing about gardening which has thus far eluded me, despite shelves full of books all called *Mr Mulch's Five-Minutes-a-Week Great Garden Guide*, then mine would be the perfect garden.

Then, last weekend I found the footling obstacle which was standing between the Gobi Desert out there and my own private Kew. For decked around the DIY centre were the parts to make my own micro-irrigation system. There were four of us weekend men standing at the massive irrigation display, turning the system's wonderful little components over in our soft hands, and I knew we were all thinking the same thing: on these display racks we had found the gardener's Rosetta Stone, the unified theory of horticultural science.

With the neat, rigid mini-tubing discreetly buried in the rich loam which my garden yearns to be, and with offshoots of micro-tubing leading to perfect miniature rotating sprayers and tiny four-litre-per-hour drippers and dinky 80-degree mist-dispensers, each feeding an individual plant with a precise amount of water and all controlled by a single turn of the tap at the back door – how could anything so sublimely complicated not be the simple answer?

Yea, and the desert shall bloom, and the land of Hammersmith shall bear the fruit of the vine and melons and dates and all sweet things: sing Hallelujah O ye children of Shepherd's Bush, and hand over the Visa card.

By the time I'd made the guess about how many 180-degree spray nozzles I'd need and what number of rigid 90-degree turns I'd have to put into the main hose, and chosen between the two dozen other items of horticultural Meccano, it was noon.

And by the time I'd got home and read the instructions which told me how many more 180-degree spray nozzles I'd need – instructions that were only accessible once I'd bought them – and driven back to the garden centre twice to change everything I'd bought the first time, and the second, it was three-ish, or five-ish with a late lunch.

By sevenish I'd laid three yards of hose and by eight I'd given up burying the hose in the rock-hard earth and just let it lie where it would in the shrivelled bushes. By nine I was ready to turn the tap.

It made the garden wet.

I don't know quite what more I'd expected it to do, of course – a wet garden being no more or less than was promised. And I knew as I watched it soak the garden in perfectly precise little squirts and sprays and dribbles that I would wake up to wet, wormy apples and dead, wet daisies and that, eventually, in a week or a month, I would ring the gardener, who would do something which involved no rigid mini-pipes and no Visa cards but probably would involve breaking into the sort of sweat that I try to avoid.

Which means, I guess, and by the identical token, that a new word-processing program won't get the novel written any more than an expensive sable brush will turn me into the water-colourist I've always believed myself to be.

I write this as if it's a sudden discovery; the truth is that I knew the moment I got the irrigation kit that a million flowers would not bloom. I accept my indolent gullibility, of course, with my usual equanimity.

But what I also know is that the people who make irrigation kits were sure that I'd turn up one day, garden dying and credit card at the ready, and that I'd spend £150 to water the garden. And that really does rankle.

The Times Magazine

25 NOVEMBER 1995
THE ECONOMY

THE MOST ACCURATE way of plotting the course of the last recession was to study the postcard-laden interiors of London phone boxes which, since the mid-Eighties, have doubled as advertising hoardings for our metropolitan hookers.

As the pound dipped against the yen and the little yuppie niche-marketing stores selling their City socks and City ties closed down, so the services offered by Bobbi and Traci and New Young Blonde In Town became ever dodgier. You knew the economy had hit bottom, if you'll pardon the expression, when sad girls with schoolgirl uniforms started asking men they'd never met to come round and beat them.

Once the girls found they could advertise for free in the centre of London, they hardly needed to congregate in the streets, which is why Soho is not the place it was. A decade ago it was still a mixture of theme-park sleaze and fancy butchers; now it's gays and huddles of drunk sales executives down from Cheadle Hulme asking the slack-faced women at the doors of the near-beer bars precisely what they'll get for their four quid.

Like the Tower devoid of Beefeaters, Disneyland without its oversized Mickeys, Soho has been stripped of its hookers. Except the other Thursday night at about eightish.

I'm walking along Shaftesbury Avenue to meet a guy who – well, whatever. A woman approaches me: twenty-eight going on forty, well turned out, dark coat, skirt short in a modest sort of way, face made up but not theatrically so. The sort of woman who might approach asking for change for the parking meter.

'I know you, don't I?' she says, beaming, and she really looks as though she does. I don't recognise her, but that doesn't mean much: there are people I've known for a decade at whom I blink confusedly when they wave at me in Sainsbury's. I try one of those distracted non-committal smiles and the beam becomes a frown.

'Or do I? Perhaps it's someone else,' she says. 'Anyway, look. I've got a little place round the corner.'

My smile gets more non-committal still. I say, 'Hnnnn. Thrp,' the way one does. 'Starts at £50,' she says. She lets her coat fall open slightly: her dress is rather less modest at the top than at the bottom.

With my usual dunderheaded *esprit d'escalier* I will realise later that the correct response is simply to walk on past like you do to collecting-tin shakers when you've already told five of their number that you gave already, but instead I say, 'Thanks very much, but really, I'm late for an appointment, not just now, thank you,' for all the world as if I hate to disappoint her, she having picked me out of a crowd because of my firm jaw line.

'Well, if you're sure, then,' she says with a sort of come-hither grimace, and I say, 'Sorry, but . . .'

And we look at each other, my dopey smile meeting her scowl, and she says, 'Well f off, then,' and marches away to find somebody else she thinks she knows.

I tell the story to the man I've gone to meet in the bar and I ask him what sociable gene led me to conspire in the fiction that the exchange was about attraction rather than commerce. He says I'm probably just a polite sort of guy and then smirks and says, 'Yeah, but you were tempted, weren't you?' I wasn't in this case, but yes, I suppose, in some purely theoretical way, I might have been something that almost comes under the heading of tempted.

We tried to work out why this was, given that had I been the late Charles Laughton dressed for *The Hunchback of Notre Dame* I would, I imagine, have been just as much a catch. More so: Laughton was worth a bob or two.

My companion doesn't know this either, but he says this is because he's never been with a prostitute. It's odd: there are

154

meant to be some 7,000 hookers working in London and I don't know a single man who admits to having used one. Me neither, but I know I'm telling the truth.

A couple of days later I see her again bumping into another man, my age, my sort of clothes, my sort of build. He looks at his watch and then sheepishly around him, and off they go, not together but in the same direction.

I don't know: perhaps she just goes for my sort of bloke.

The Times Magazine

2 MARCH 1996

ORDINARY PEOPLE

WE DIAMONDS HAVE never been snobs – people of our breeding so rarely are – but there are times I feel less than well disposed towards the smart-alec British Rail apparatchik who invented the Weekend First fare, which, for an extra fiver, lets any old traveller transfer from the guard's van to the comfy seats.

Because here I am, almost a double for one of the smug, bespectacled exec types who takes the train whenever there happens to be a British Rail first-class *Executive Magazine* photographer around, typing away on the laptop somewhere south of Manchester, when two lads come and sit opposite me, ignoring completely the special pull-out supplement on the Azerbaijani economic miracle which I've spread over the other three seats by way of a multiple seat reservation.

'What game you playing, then?' one of them says after a minute or so.

It's not a game, I say. I'm writing something.

'You a writer, then?' the other one says.

I don't really know why I should feel it necessary to initiate them in my campaign to stop journalists calling themselves writers, but I tell him that no, I'm a journalist. I'm writing for a newspaper.

They pause for a minute.

'Go on, then – write something about us, then.'

I look up. What about you?

'I dunno. Anything. Get us names in the paper. Go on.'

They are big lads, severe haircuts, mortgageable training

shoes, 300-quid parkas, with open cans of beer between their knees, and spares in the little polythene holders next to them. I give them a look that is meant to suggest that, God knows, if it were just up to me I'd have them all over the front pages, but you know how picky editors are, and go back to typing.

They mistranslate the look, although I'm not quite sure what their mistranslation is. They carry on pestering away in a sort of newspaperish equivalent of jumping up and down behind the political correspondent who's trying to say his piece into the TV camera, as if by force of tipsy will our conversation will put them in print.

'Go on, write something about us.'

What can I tell them? That I don't know anything about them? That 'Wilmslow Two Found Drinking Carlsberg on InterCity' is not a story? But why should they believe me? For as long as there have been tabloids, there have been news stories in them which might just as well have appeared under the headline 'Journalist Finds Two Men in Right Place at Right Time' – stories about ordinary people doing ordinary things, which just happen to have come to the attention of the press.

Perhaps it's not a news story they're after, though; perhaps they think they could appear in the features pages, their surnames dropped for the sake of anonymity, telling all about sex in the suburbs or the horror which is Carlsberg addiction.

Or, then again, maybe I'm being patronising. Perhaps these two are broadsheet readers. After all, there's at least one serious-minded paper which specialises in sending sassy young journalists out to spend twelve hours in a launderette or a motorway service station, seeing what something called real life looks like – as if we can only ever know that life filtered through a shorthand notebook.

Either way, they seem not to understand any connection between newspapers and news. As they seem to understand it, newspapers aren't there to connect our lives to those of our rulers, to describe the most current condition of our world. Newspapers, they have learnt, are simply daily lists of interesting but random things: facts, rants, opinions, pictures and, above all, names.

Indeed, every properly trained journalist starts life on a local weekly, where the trick is to attach as many local names to each wedding, funeral, Rotary club meeting or car crash as possible. Perhaps those two think journalists are the secular equivalent of those Buddhist monks who spend their lives writing all the possible names of God into ledgers, and that journalism's job will be finished when every name has been consigned to print.

They get off the train at Stafford. Just before they go they try again. 'Go on, mate. Why not? Go on. Put us in your paper.'

So I did.

The Times Magazine

14 September 1996

I THOUGHT I HAD CANCER

IT'S EASY FOR me to say, of course, now that I've spent a couple of days on BUPA's money tramping around the back alleys of Harley Street offering up sundry fluids to transient Australian nurses making up their Munich Bierfest cash with a spot of casual cytology, but there is a certain sort of liberation in learning one might have cancer.

Suddenly, unbidden, amid the throbbing-all-over, body-hugging panic, appeared the thought that I could forget the common courtesies for a while. I could stop worrying about returning calls, getting things done on time, doing my citizenly duty. People, I knew, would understand.

One doesn't like to take liberties with one's own mortal fear, but I felt I could phone up the Inland Revenue or the VAT and say, look, hold on for a while on the outstanding few thousands will you guys? It's just that I have cancer.

I practised the last three words in my head a few times. A sad smile? A tremor in the voice? A pause before the last, drastic word? But no, I thought: too dramatic, too affected, too demanding of the right response. But either way, what could the tax people say? When I was still potentially cancerous I imagined them breaking down and cancelling the debt; now I realise that the one group the Revenue would be particularly keen to keep in touch with are those ingrates who are in danger of pegging it before the money's paid in full.

Cancer has a special place in every hypochondriac's demonology because it's the one that gives you a chance to be smug, to reap the rewards of all those years of knowing it had to happen some day. Our only other worry, whatever we say, is the sudden massive heart attack which is, well, too *sudden* to capitalise on.

But the real fear, I discovered – and call me the Enlightenment's Mr Slowcoach if you must – is not dying itself, but dying and going to hell. Sure, I know that for we secular types hell is only an irrational rationalisation for an otherwise inexplicable fear of dying, but the terror is much the same. As the impossible death becomes a mad possibility, so do all the other impossibilities, including the fiery brimstone-ish ones, and it seems rationality doesn't cut it when it comes to subconscious terrors brought to the surface in a doctor's surgery.

And all the while that you're being terrified, you have to go for tests and tests and tests because BUPA is the very reverse of the NHS. Go to the NHS with a lump on your neck and they'll give you a blood test and then, when the results of that's come through, put you on the list for the cytologist and when the cytologist's done you'll queue for days or weeks, depending on which point in the financial year you choose to have the lump, and eventually you'll get an answer.

BUPA gives you a cheerful Harley Street specialist the day after tomorrow. And he sends you, that very afternoon, to the waiting rooms of blood-testing centres and Cat-scan installations, where the teenage children of visiting Arab sheikhs are looking through the rural property sections of *Country Life* and laughing, and where chic nurses in gleaming uniforms dispense invoices from behind little notices listing the credit cards that are acceptable and home laser-printed warnings that cheques will only be accepted up to the amount on the guarantee card, like some high-rent car workshop.

But there is one test, the definitive test, and that can't be arranged for a week, during which time we perform a thousand small acts of exegesis on every possible intonation of every phrase the doctor used, and by the end of the week I know I have a Hodgkin's lymphoma at the very least because why would BUPA stump up this sort of money to test for a relatively unusual form of cyst?

Which is, it turns out, what I have. A week of antibiotics

and then a couple of nights in hospital while they cut it out.

Well, whew! (And I speak now as one who knows what whew! looks like from the inside.) But just as that tiny thought of liberation crept in alongside the terror, so alongside the relief is an even tinier thought of having been cheated of my own nemesis. It is, I imagine, the effect of having lost one's immediate sense of mortality while knowing that one's immortality will never be returned.

The Times Magazine

25 JANUARY 1997

MY HASSIDIC PROBLEM

I DON'T KNOW why I have any problem other than a purely intellectual one with the Hassidim; the part of London where I grew up was Hassid City and on high days Springfield Park was black with them all walking down to the River Lea.

Or, at least, I don't know where my original problem comes from. I can date my modern problem with them quite precisely.

A while ago my father's computer broke. It was an ancient thing, and I hunted through the computer magazines until I found somewhere which promised it could fix any computer ever built. The shop was in the east London land of my fathers and at the main desk sat a youngish man in fur-trimmed hat and what Dickens referred to as side-locks.

He looked at the computer and told me it would be ready on Thursday. Six months later they'd rebuilt the computer and it sat on the man's desk while the man beamed at me.

'What do I owe you?' I said.

He looked at me and pursed his lips. His brother came and joined him. 'You're Jewish, no?' said his brother.

'I'm Jewish, yes,' I said.

'So when did you last say the *Shema*?' The *Shema* is your basic everyday confession of Jewish faith, the Jewish equivalent of the Lord's Prayer. There are various Hassidic groups who take particularly seriously the divine injunction to perform *mitzvah*s – obligations, *inter alia*, to perform meritorious deeds which are collected like so many heavenly Air Miles to be cashed in come the Last Trump. Bringing the lapsed back into the flock, even to the extent of getting him to recite the *Shema*, counts as a *mitzvah*.

The last time I said the *Shema*, I told him, I was eleven and I learnt it, phonetically rather than in Hebrew, because the local youth club with the best girls was next door to a synagogue and its youth leader demanded that all newcomers be able to recite the prayer.

'OK. Here's what we do. You say the *Shema*, we call it quits.'

Fair deal. I slapped my hand on my head for want of a *yarmulke* and started. '*Shema y'Israel . . .*' I got as far as '*echod*' at the end of the second line, and then corpsed.

There was a pause.

'OK. No problem,' said the man. 'Shlomo!' he called up the stairs. An elderly man hobbled down the staircase holding an eight-foot by four-sheet of hardboard. He propped it against the desk. It was the Hebrew equivalent of those curtains which drop down at the back of pantomime stages with the words of 'I've Got a Lovely Bunch of Coconuts' to help the audience along.

'I'm sorry,' I said, and felt it. 'I don't read Hebrew.'

'No problem,' said the man. 'Shlomo . . .'

The elderly man turned the hardboard sheet around. On the other side were the words of the *Shema* written in phonetic English.

I started again.

'Shema y'Israel . . .'

They let me get halfway through the prayer book before they stopped me.

'Not with the hand,' said the man. 'You got a *koppel*?' That I should have forgotten the *Shema* and be unable to speak Hebrew – and yet still carry a *yarmulke* with me was taking unworldliness a bit far. No. I didn't have one.

'Shlomo . . .'

Shlomo carefully removed his fur-trimmed hat, stroked the *yarmulke* beneath it and passed the hat to me. I grimaced. The man looked at me. I put it on.

This time I got almost all the way through before he stopped me. 'No. You can't do it that way. Shlomo – the *tefillin*.'

Tefillin are phylacteries: leather boxes containing the small print of the contract between God and Moses, and which the devout bind around their heads and forearms from time to time.

I wanted to say, Stop! Whatever the computer costs, I'll pay. This is wrong. This is not who I am, and you know this is not who I am, and yet here you are, pushing your luck for the sake of a *mitzvah*, and here I am pushing my luck for the sake of a free computer repair.

But I didn't stop. I rattled through the prayer and whipped off the hat and the phylacteries, and grabbed the computer.

As I ran out I glanced at the sundry West Indians, Irishmen and others who made up the rest of the repair company, but they all had their heads down at the other end of the office. They'd seen it before.

The Times Magazine

1 FEBRUARY 1997

THE SECRETS OF NOSTRADAMUS

A TELEOLOGIST, EVER wise after an event, is a man who can do yesterday's newspaper crossword puzzle, but only when he's got today's solution in front of him.

He'll smirk and tell you that of course he knew the answers all along, show you just why each clue leads to its particular word and tell you that, actually he is a world authority on crossword puzzles.

The best teleologists of all, which is to say those who make a living from their skill, are the members of the Nostradamus club.

In the middle of the sixteenth century Michel de Nostradame, astrologer and physician, wrote and published a book on jam-making and, more famously, 1,000 quatrains claiming to predict – or, as David Ovason has it, prevision – the future. The jam book has been forgotten, but for the more than 400 years since Nostradamus's death academics, fellow seers, writers of popular occultism and assorted con merchants have been arguing about precisely what those provisions were.

Their teleological trick is to identify, using 20–20 hindsight, those things Nostradamus foretold in what was then his future and has since become our past. But the paradox of his prophesies is that they are so garbled that they only become prophesies once they have happened.

The problem is that Nostradamus wrote neither in French nor in his local Provençal dialect, nor either of the two classical languages, but in a sort of random mixture of the four – a *scabreux* language, as he candidly described it. And since his death numerous experts have come along to explain that they are the first to understand Nostradamus's language and thus the first to give the correct interpretation of his prophesies.

Interpretation isn't simply a matter of translating his quatrains into a modern language, as even when translated they are apparently meaningless. To find their true sense the teleologist must use anagrams, complicated sums, or deduce the meaning using metaphor.

The problem with metaphor, though, is that it is such a vague instrument. This is why quatrain X.22, for instance, has been translated at various times, with equal certainty, as foretelling the beheading of Charles I, the abdication of Edward VIII and the divorce of Charles and Diana.

It reads: For not wishing to consent to the divorce,/Which afterwards will be recognised as unworthy,/The King of the Isles will be driven out by force,/Put in his place one who has no sign of Kingship.

That there have been so many 'first correct' interpretations is, in itself, an inexplicable paradox. For if each new expert is the first to explain how accurate Nostradamus's predictions are, then it follows that his predecessor's translations were inaccurate. This, then, begs the question as to why a book of inaccurate prophesies has been considered so remarkably accurate for so long.

David Ovason is the latest to claim the one true interpretation – unfortunately in a ponderous, repetitive and pompous way. His claim is based not on a greater knowledge of anagram or metaphor, but on a deeper understanding of the Green language – a tongue unknown to any linguist, but understood in 'astro-alchemy'.

The basis of the Green language is that secret words and meanings are hidden away in other words. Thus, according to the French speaker, Reynard means 'fox'. And, according to the fluent Green speakers, the word hides two other words – reign meaning 'king' and art meaning, well, art.

Thus a Green speaker coming across Reynard in a Nostradamus quatrain will understand that we are talking about a man skilled in the art of kingship.

Using this language Ovason, a teacher of astrology, proves – and I use the word very loosely – that Nostradamus could predict the planetary conjunctions. If you know when the planets were in any particular conjunction you can look below them, see what was going on in Earth and tie the quatrain to a particular prediction.

As David Ovason freely admits: 'Nostradamus wrote predictions which were totally incomprehensible prior to the events prophesied.' Given the broad sweep of history it would be amazing if over 500 years he didn't have some lucky hits. Although, as the American commentator Bergen Evans wrote in 1955: 'Nostradamus's rate of success is considerably below what he would have obtained by flipping a coin.'

Ovason seems to have shortened the odds a little, however, by picking his quatrains carefully. Of the full 1,000, Ovason gives us precise details of fewer than seventy of them, and even here he has to work hard to make them fit.

To give him his due, Ovason works hard even when the meaning is apparently obvious. When Nostradamus seems to specify July 1999 for some apocalyptic event, Ovason proves he actually means 2087. A glimpse at part of his equation is thus: 'If we subtract 28 years from 4005 we obtain 3977. This is a numerological anagram for 3797 . . .' From this you can see how hard he works to make fact fit half-baked theory.

Is Ovason right? I have subjected his own name to the Green technique and discovered that Ovason breaks down into ova, or egg, and son, which is the French for sound. Ovason, therefore, becomes 'egg sound', and the sound an egg makes is that of cracking. Thus the words Ovason and crackers are, in Green language, entirely cognate.

Daily Mail

Review of *The Secrets of Nostradamus* by David Ovason (Century, 1997)

8 MARCH 1997

THINGS YOU DIDN'T KNOW
ABOUT ARTHROPODS

WE WERE AT the Natural History Museum, not because we wanted to see anything natural or learn its history, but because we'd been invited to a birthday party. The Natural History Museum Tandoori Grill-a-GoGo is where you go for great parties nowadays: they shove a couple of pteranodons into a corner and pack away the odd intrusive triceratops and put out the tables, unless it's a cocktail party, in which case you get to lean against a stuffed blue whale while you grind the Twiglets underfoot.

It's not just the Natural History Museum: all London's great museums have turned themselves into sprauncy venues for book launches and birthday parties in which the skeletal remains of the Mesozoic period serve not as *memento mori* to our own species, but as clever backdrops to the canapés and the chatter.

I'm not saying it's wrong, not least because it really was a very good party, but standing in as a banqueting suite is somehow below the old institution's natural dignity – assuming, that is, that learning still has some dignity.

Which is not to say that the museums don't still serve some vague educational function during the partyless days, and we found ourselves wandering into an exhibition of a hundred things you didn't know about arthropods. Everything was displayed in that modern way that museums have – the way which says, 'Look, we curators are happening people. We understand that if we said we had a room full of arthropods with labels telling you what they were like, well like as not you'd be off, er, grooving in the discotheque or whatever it is. So what we've done is to hire somebody who speaks fluent Dim-ese to help us pretend that this is nothing to do with personal enrichment but is a rather pleasant video-game arcade.'

The result is that herbivores and carnivores have become members of new taxonomies to which we happening people can so easily relate: they are labelled 'Vegetarians' and 'Meat-Eaters' like so many little Linda McCartneys or Jonathan Meadeses scuttling around the forest floor.

But more lip-pursingly annoying still are the headings on the explanatory notes at each exhibit. Over the praying mantis is a sign saying 'Getting to Grips' and over some other arthropod is another reading 'Up for Grabs'.

I spent a minute trying to work out what the resonances were until it occurred to me that these weren't museum labels: they were tabloid newspaper headlines. Yes: even our noblest museums have fallen foul of that most insidious late-twentieth-century scourge – the newspaperisation of everything.

It's not just that headline phrases like 'Shock Horror!' have entered the language, or that people routinely use hyperbolic newspaper words – terror, shame, crisis – to describe events which are less than terrifying, shameful or critical, but that so many non-journalists find the conventions and metaphors of the newsdesk so convenient a way of doing their job.

Look at the number of ads which rely on the newspaper headline to make their point, or the regularity with which I get calls from teachers who want help with turning history or geography lessons into class newspapers. Look how often the broadcast media use newspaper experts rather than the first-principle experts to whom journalists go for their facts.

I can't complain, of course, for the greater the incursion of the press into our general culture, the greater the chance the press – with me as a member of it – has of staving off TV and radio as the prime media.

But I only realised the extent to which the press serves as a common focus when I got an e-mail from a man complaining that a column I wrote the other week was a coded message about him. In fact, the man has for some time now been flooding the Internet with messages saying that the press is devoted to harassing him with coded messages and that Bernard Levin's writings on Wagner are in fact writings on him.

My correspondent is quite open about the fact that he's been diagnosed as a schizophrenic, and when I explained that the column wasn't about him at all he sent me a sweet message explaining that sometimes his illness got the better of him, but it struck me that ten or twenty years ago anyone with a persecution complex would have looked elsewhere to find the source of his persecution.

The Times Magazine

5 APRIL 1997

IT'S EVERYWHERE

I AM SITTING in a day room in St George's Hospital in Tooting.

I'd intended starting this on a more impressive note of pathos: 'I'm lying in my hospital bed waiting for the pill which will allow me to deal less anxiously with the fact that tomorrow a man will come and knock me out and carve slices out of my neck, which he'll inspect for malignancy,' but a conceited traffic accident victim or selfishly relapsing cancer patient sneaked in and took the bed – my bed – and so, for some hours, I've been shuttled from one day room to another, and now it's no longer even day.

At least it's given me a chance to study the hospital's collection of discreet *memento mori*. It's not just the leaflets from the local council posted around the place telling you, so tastefully, how to register a death, or the instructions on how to get hold of the emergency priest or rabbi when the moment comes. It's everywhere.

The reception area is piled with old glossy magazines, each one especially selected to remind you of what the worst-case scenario is about hospitals – and, while you're here, the only-case scenario about life generally. 'When You've Got to Go . . .', a piece on weekend breaks in *Country Life* is headlined, and 'Dead Reckoning', an article on graveyard photography in *Amateur Photography*. The headlines leap out of pieces on the mundanities of travel and cooking and wine: 'A Grave Situation', 'No Hope of Return', 'Heaven Can't Wait'.

News update: they've just told me there is a bed after all.

True, it's so far from the hospital's ear, nose and throat sector that they might have to reschedule the operation, but it's a bed. On a public ward. And I feel so crass doing the 'What the hell do I pay BUPA all that money for if I can't have a room to myself' schtick in front of a row of patients who have probably been hanging around for months on waiting lists hoping to get a bed in the NHS lottery.

But anger overcomes crassness and so I've just had one of those Californian arguments with the woman in charge of beds, the sort where I say I realise it's not your fault, but you must understand I'm very angry and there's nobody else around to shout at, and where she says that she appreciates my anger, and she is hearing my shouting, but there is nothing really that she can do.

And just before she goes, she smiles in that soft nursish way and says she is sure everything will be all right. It's easy for her to say: she'll be sleeping in her own bed tonight.

That's what everyone says. I phone up friends and say, Look, you remember that lump on my neck? Well, they're cutting it out and the doctor says he wants to take a look around, just to see what's in there, rather like a police diver uses the phrase just before he goes over the edge of the dinghy into the murky and body-ridden lake. And my friends say, 'Hey, don't worry. It'll be fine. I know it'll be fine.' Which is what we all say when we're not quite sure what the right thing to say is.

It would be reassuring if my friends were surgeons, or nurses, or even pharmacists, but they're journalists and radio producers and magazine editors, and what they don't know about surgery would fill two or three large medical libraries. How do they know it will be fine, that the lump is just one of those lumps you get from time to time? Not even the surgeon knows that.

I can't even put it down to my normal hypochondria. Hypochondria usually comes in two varieties. The chronic version, which turns every twinge into a cardiac event, every spot into a melanoma, every cold into pneumonia, is the worse because of the not knowing. By comparison, the acute version, in which a real doctor with a real medical degree tells you that you do have some actual minor illness and that you can legitimately look ill when you tell people about it in the pub, is, in its way, rather cheering.

But this is beyond those conditions. Nobody can tell me that the fear of being put under for a couple of hours while they cut your neck open is an irrational one.

The pill is taking hold. I shall go to bed now. A public bed in a public ward, but one with clean sheets and surrounded by calm nurses who accept that men who are about to go under the knife get angry. And frightened. Because while BUPA covers most contingencies, it doesn't cover fear.

The Times Magazine

12 April 1997

NOT THE REAL ME

THE ME YOU meet here isn't the real me. He looks much the same as the real me, has the same number of wives and children, combines wit and witlessness in roughly the same proportions, has lived much the same life in many of the same places, but you will understand that if each week I were to deliver to you my life unpasteurised and absolutely as I experience it then that life would be unlivable.

There are, I know, domestic columnists around whose relationship with their partners, their parents, their cleaners and other walk-on characters is so mature – or possibly immature – that they can report every detail of it unfiltered for public inspection and be on speaking terms with their subjects at the end of the exercise. Not me. The me you see here is a sort of parallel me, picking and choosing the details which will best make the point, changing names or job titles out of a sense of propriety or social cowardice, baring a virtual soul and taking risks only where no risk really exists.

Until last week.

Six months or so ago I wrote about the lump in my neck. I started the piece with a disingenuous reference to an illness which might or might not turn out to be something nasty, and finished it with a smug punchline which, looking back at it now, sneered at anyone who might have been worrying for 800 words worth of affected angst whether they were watching a man whose head was about to clunk insensate on to the keyboard.

And then last week I tried the trick again. I'm not quite sure what I wrote because I dispatched the words only a couple of days ago, and because I really did write it in the hospital ward I don't have the piece to hand. But I seem to remember leaving my readers with unanswered questions in the full expectation that at the end of some inconsequential column or another this week I'd note that, by the way, and thanks for asking, I came round from the operation and everything was fine. I was frightened, sure, but the fear I wrote about was, I now know, the ersatz version which one knows will pass with the cause.

At eight p.m. on the night I am writing this the consultant phoned up with the bad news, and what do you know? I had cancer all along. And have it still. The hubris-hating gods, it seems, read *The Times* too.

So here's my problem. Well, not my real problem, which is that I have cancer and may expire before the date printed on the packet, but my columnar problem.

Cancer is a word of such immense potency that one has to be careful how one uses it in a column. I know the disease is nothing special: people die of it all the time and many more live with, and through, cancer, and I may well be one of the latter. I won't know for certain until they've scanned me next week and carved some random bits out of my throat for inspection, one of the many crass jokes of cancer being that in the early stages the diagnosis is more physically painful than the disease itself.

The question is this: is it appropriate to write about one's own cancer in a jaunty weekend column? Of course, there's no guarantee that I'll be able to keep up the jauntiness, especially as the various alternative treatments have the side-effect, says my doctor, of 'making you feel a bit miserable'.

So can I keep the jauntiness up under radiotherapy or, worse, if they tell me I've got only another few dozens columns left in me? Should I keep it up?

I am suddenly very conscious of how I look sitting here. Normally any smugness or bravado or megalomania I exhibit in this space and in my parallel persona doesn't worry me too much: claiming a regular dozen square inches in the country's foremost paper – the paper, after all, the gods read – doesn't make much sense if you're not prepared to be those things.

This is a personal column: I can't just pretend that the event which is currently informing everything I think or do doesn't exist. But if the cancer turns out to be curable don't I risk sounding smugger than ever? And if it doesn't – well, what sort of maudlin is that?

Normally I try to address any qualms I have about what I'm about to write before I sit down to write it. This time, I'm sorry, I can't. There you are: the truth, at last.

The Times Magazine

19 April 1997

THINGS ARE SO-SO

YOU GET TO a certain age, you assume you've got a handle on most of social intercourse's more likely eventualities. After a few false starts you've learnt how to do sending the meal back, dropping the girlfriend, getting through the job interview, making the marriage proposal, and you think you've got it taped. And then one day some new circumstance pitches up and you realise that you're not, after all, living the life you thought you were living, and that there are some quite basic exchanges you don't know how to do.

A friend phones up and asks, as is the way of these things, how I am. Sometimes I forget how I am. I say: 'Fine, and you?' and then I have to backtrack, because of course I'm not fine. So I say, 'Actually, I say that, I say I'm fine, but, well, I've got cancer.'

What else can you say? You can't build up to it slowly – 'I'm ill. No, not a cold, really ill. No, worse than flu. No, no; better than Aids but worse than flu. OK, two syllables . . .' – or drop it casually into the conversation: 'Things? Things are so-so, you know? I got the new computer, and somebody broke the car window and nicked the stereo, and I've got throat cancer, and we thought of going to see *Jerry Maguire*, but . . .'

So I just say I've got cancer. For the first few days I said it as often as I could because I still didn't quite believe it. We would sit in the consultant's office surrounded by chatty leaflets on nausea in chemotherapy and say to each other, 'What are we doing here?' But now, a ten-day lifetime into it

177

all, I am used to it, and I know that when I say cancer what they hear me say is that I'm about to die.

Which, it turns out, I'm probably not.

My carcinoma is squamous, which means not only that it wins high points on the Scrabble board but that it's as miserable a thing as one can have and yet bear the name cancer still. It is low-grade, says my GP; non-aggressive says the hospital; and, my favourite this, according to a medical friend who swears it's a kosher medical term, indolent. I have a 92 per cent chance of living for ten years, says one of the thousands of pages on the Internet devoted to cancer. At last: a use for the Internet! Who'd have guessed?

It will involve six weeks of daily radiotherapy, the loss of half my salivatory system, a few nasty symptoms which, says the doctor, will make me feel 'miserable', regular check-ups for years to come and a temporary hiatus in my broadcasting career. In fact, I thought I could even get away with broadcasting until I mistakenly did an episode of the *News Quiz* the day after a painful biopsy and finished up sounding like the love child of Janet Street-Porter and Jack Ashley MP. Some or all of which is what I tell those who ask how things are going. 'Yes,' they say, 'I'm sure you're going to be OK,' but they don't really believe it. Or at least they do believe it, but it doesn't really square with what they know – what we all know – about cancer. Even the doctors fall for the word's more obvious associations. The morning after the consultant had phoned with the bad news, I turned up at the hospital to hear the small print read out. 'I've got cancer then,' I said. 'Yes,' the consultant said, and paused. 'I'm sorry,' and he said that sorry with the downcast face of someone who is giving the worst news – even though the news he had to give was that the chances were that I would go through eight weeks of misery and emerge at the other end with little more than some slight sunburn where the radiotherapy had done its stuff. Medicine has, as they say, made great strides (as in 'Great strides, Doctor! Love the turn-ups!') and much cancer is curable. But even if the prognosis has changed, the word hasn't. And much as I've learnt about cancer over the past couple of weeks, I'm still a sucker for its potency. I get to the end of the explanation of how this isn't quite as bad a deal as the phrase 'I've got cancer' suggests and, mollified, the voice at the other end of the phone says, 'Well that's all right then.' And I find myself saying, well, no: it's still cancer. Real cancer. If I'm stuck with a stigmatised disease, the least I can do is to accept the sympathy that should go with it.

The Times Magazine

14 JUNE 1997

SELLING ROSES ON THE

CROMWELL ROAD

THERE IS A man who patrols the central reservation of the Cromwell Road in Earls Court with roses in a bucket. A sign on the bucket says they're two quid the bunch, which seems cheap even for roses as limp and tawdry as his. He looks like a Serb: somebody once told me that the traffic-jam rose-selling game in London is run by Bosnian Serbs and that it's a cover for something nasty, although I can't remember what it's meant to be a cover for or, come to that, imagine what it could be a cover for.

Each day I drive for a mile or so along this sclerotic west London artery and, as I wait in the fifteen-minute queue for the filter-lane lights to change and let me take the turn towards the hospital in Fulham, I watch him shuffling his floral sentry duty up and down the concrete isle, proffering his sad, wilting bunches in their unlikely, hot-house, lipstick colours at the drivers, and smiling a sad, wilting smile as they shake their heads and look the other way.

In six weeks I have yet to see him sell a single rose. I must have watched him for getting on for ten hours in total during what must be the period when home-going men are most likely to be in the market for a guilt-cancelling rose or two. And I can't work out why he carries on doing it, why, after two months, he hasn't realised what every driver who passes him realises, which is that there is no market for roses on the Cromwell Road.

I keep on thinking that I should buy a bunch, to cheer him up, but that would be unfair to both of us. Unfair to me because I'd have a bunch of wilting cerise roses which I wouldn't dare give to any woman I know, and unfair to him because I wouldn't want to give him the impression that there might, after all, be a future for his business when so obviously there isn't.

Tomorrow, though, it will be too late, for I will have stopped being a Cromwell Road commuter. By the time you read this I shall have been zapped for the last time. It's been just over two months since I mentioned here that I was about to go under the knife and just under two months since I shared with you the surprise of what that knife had discovered. In between then and now I have sat down at the start of each week and tried to work out what I wanted to say, or could usefully say about cancer that I hadn't said the week before.

Protracted illness has so little by way of plot, doesn't it? Yes, there's the run-up to it, and one day I hope there will be a proper dénouement, and there are odd days of new activity, but in between there is only disease's unbreakable iteration.

Yes, there is also – as I mentioned the other week – the tedium of the treatment, but that's not the problem. Rather, it's that what I really want to do is that which a columnist is bound not to do: write precisely the same thing every week.

I don't mean something like the same thing, or a variant of what I said last week, but exactly the same thing. Each week I want to start, 'What stale hell is this?' I want to write that my neck hurts and I can't taste anything and food makes me retch, and that I'm still scared much of the time, but these aren't statements which common journalistic courtesy allows you to make more than once.

Illness has its ups and downs, its good days and its bad, but the big picture is one of relentlessness, of waking up every morning and it still being there. Each week I want to write, 'You know how I said last week that even the water tastes of battery acid? Well, it still tastes of battery acid. And you know what? Next week, and probably the week after that, it will taste of battery acid and I'll want to tell you about it again.'

It is the iteration rather than the pain itself which makes ill people crotchety. It is being in that state where you want people to ask how you are so that you can glower at them and tell them that you're just the same as you were last time they asked, thanks very much.

There you are: I promised not to moan, and I've moaned. It could, I know, be worse. I could be not selling roses on the Cromwell Road.

The Times Magazine

12 JULY 1997

NANNYDOM

THERE NOW FOLLOWS a break in normal transmission while they decide whether I'm cured or not. For which, thank God, and not least because the nanny gave notice last week and all bets, oncological and otherwise, are off until we've replaced her.

In fact, I say the nanny, but we've never called her that. We call her by her name and hope people will get the contextual point; and she describes herself with a raised eyebrow as 'You know, the nanny or whatever,' which more or less describes the state of liberal angst which goes with nanny ownership among the non-employing classes who suddenly discover they've got a Victorian complement of staff, what with cleaning ladies turning up so regularly they become transmogrified into housekeepers, and men who once appeared for an afternoon to help get the garden into shape now coming on a regular basis. It's only a matter of time before we have a bloke in striped trousers at the front door asking who should he say is calling.

But meanwhile we have the nanny problem, which involves the subsidiary problem of admitting to nannydom. It wouldn't be a problem were it not for the friends who manage to spit the word 'nanny' in that supercilious way that suggests we've sent the kids off to boarding kennels until they've passed their driving tests. Given that most of said friends drop off their children in the dank basements of Kilburn child-minders while they're off middle-managing, this is a bit rich.

The only advantage of child-minding is that at least you

never know if your child is being minded by a psychopath, while the evidence of a psychopathic nanny is all around you. We took on a giantess of a New Zealander called Tatyana who came on like a real person at her interview then revealed her true spookiness over the next two weeks while we huddled in corners having whispered conversations about what it was that was so disturbing about her, other than her habit of up-ending the fridge and tipping the contents down her throat.

In fact, we only discovered how spooky she was after she'd left and our two-year-old daughter started dropping references to the monsters who lived in our garden and who would eat her unless she sat quietly while *The Lion King* was on the television.

But sacking nannies, and especially the live-in Antipodean versions, is as problematic as employing them. You phone up the agency and tell them that actually things aren't working out, no absolutely nothing major, just a personality clash sort of thing, and Tatyana disappears for a couple of afternoons to see if other couples can spot her psychopathy, and eventually a couple phone to say, 'We've just interviewed Tatyana and she seems super. How have you found her?' to which you want to answer, well, we just looked in the larder and there she was with her mouth round a family-sized packet of digestives and the bread knife in her hand. But you can't.

Because, if you tell the truth about the noises coming from her room, and the phone bill and the missing Calpol, they'll never take her off your hands. And so you make ambivalent noises about tidiness and punctuality and sidestep the question about discipline and feel guilty when a couple of days later she tells you that she's got the great new job with these super people. But not as guilty as you do when two weeks later you hear on the west London grapevine that Tatyana climaxed a week of spookiness by waiting until her new employer was serving the soup course to her new boss and eating a whole tray of the lamb chops which were to follow.

Tomorrow we start on the nightmare of interviewing, and this time we've decided no more Mr and Mrs Nice Guy. We don't want Antipodeans who have been told in some Christchurch student pub that you can work your cushy way round Europe changing nappies, and we don't want sad-faced girls who take up more space in the house than the rest of us put together, and most of all we don't want psychopaths.

Above all, we want somebody who – and call me soft if you like – when the time comes to get rid of her, we can pass on to the next set of suckers with an easy conscience.

The Times Magazine

30 AUGUST 1997

IATROGENESIS

THERE IS NO medical concept that the smug woodbark pushers and the om-chanters like better than iatrogenic illness, said illness being that brought upon patients by doctors in their attempt to cure whatever the opposite of iatrogenic illness is. Iatrogenic illness tells the energy-line followers and the bump-diviners that orthodox medicine doesn't have all the answers, which is fine with them because energy-line following and bump-divining doesn't have any of the answers at all, and in the slapdash calculus of alternative medicine some answers and no answers amount to much the same thing.

In fact, many of those who have written to suggest I steer clear of some of the nastier slash-and-burn regimens have used iatrogenic illness as the big argument, and I'd happily take their point if to the statistics on the number of people who have picked up nasty illnesses in hospitals they'd attach the number who had survived cancer without recourse to the medical orthodoxy.

All of which I could write with greater conviction if I wasn't in something of an ongoing iatrogenic situation myself.

I woke up at two in the morning the other night knowing I was about to die. I'm not talking panic-attack whimsy here: as I slept my post-operative windpipe filled with scar tissue and a gallon of phlegmy gunk and stopped piping wind. The ambulance turned up some minutes after I'd passed from gasping-beached-fish stage to unconsciousness and the next thing I knew was that I was coming round in the local A and E department attached to some more tubes.

The next day they ambulanced me to my home hospital, where they put me under for the fifth time, shoved a plastic pipe into a hole in my throat and gave me back my old bed for a few days while the antibiotics and the steroids dealt with the gunk and the swelling. I breathe again, but the tracheostomy stays in at least until they see how my throat reacts to the iatrogenic trauma which a second course of radiotherapy will offer.

I am home and resting, but what I am resting from is not cancer. I am resting from an illness caused by an illness caused by curing cancer. My irritating daily domestic regimes – cleaning and swapping tracheostomy inner tubes, painting my gums with fluoride, filling little sprays with saline solution – have nothing to do with cancer but are to support cancer's care.

In fact, I no longer really have any sense of being a cancer patient. The cancer has taken on a hermetic existence and will be cured, or not, by the radiotherapy. I have, perched above the cancer, a series of iatrogenic complaints, all of which I accept as part of the deal I make with the orthodoxy but which upset me nonetheless.

The illness which most upsets me is that which leaves me coughing and spluttering, unable to eat properly, talking as if . . .

Actually, I'm not quite sure as if what. I picked up a cab in front of the hospital when I left the other day and when I tried to tell the cabby where I wanted to go all I got was a series of clicks and hisses. But I'd prepared myself: from my pocket I produced a piece of paper on which I'd written my home address. He nodded and we set off in silence. Outside my front door the clock showed £8: I passed across a tenner.

'No,' he said.

I honked and waved the note at him.

'No. I don't want it.'

He looked at me miserably. This was his act of charity. I threw the money down next to his seat. He picked it up, came round and pushed it into a carrier bag I was holding.

'No,' he said again, and drove off, angry with my ungraciousness.

Here I was, hale apart from the small portion between my nose and my neck, cabbing it to a reasonable home in a reasonable part of town. And what did he see? I really don't know. A man coming home from the cancer ward to die? A mute who, by that definition alone, must need the money?

There have been some depressing moments in the past months but none quite so depressing as standing on the pavement watching the cabby drive away without my money, pitying me for my iatrogenesis.

The Times Magazine

13 September 1997

NOT MYSELF

When I tell you that I am not myself at the moment I don't mean merely that I am in a state of discomfort but that I really am not me: I am somebody else. Precisely, I am currently a little old man who I imagine is called Albert or Norman or George.

Certainly I am little, or at least littler than I ever have been in my adult life.

Have you ever lost weight? I don't mean the few pounds which you couldn't face hanging over the top of your bathing trunks, or the wobbly stone that lingered postpartum, but I mean real weight, whole chunks of corporation, enough spare body to make another small person.

At my chubby and pre-cancerous high point I weighed a few ounces more than fifteen stone; yesterday I weighed in at something incomprehensibly metric, which turns out to be eleven stone and a bit. By my reckoning, I have lost a leg-and-a-half's worth of me.

An old leg-and-a-half's worth, at that, a leg-and-a-half's worth from the days when my thigh still had its familiar triangular cross section and my calf bulged over the top of my sock. Now I look in the mirror and there is a different man looking back, a stranger whose stick legs drop away from his tiny rump, whose wiry arms are only muscle and bone, a man with very little belly to speak of.

I have the New Age body that I always associate with the sort of men who dress in drawstring trousers, run primal scream therapy sessions in north London and tell you that

189

they've never felt healthier since they went fruitarian in '87.

The weight loss came as a surprise. Not the loss itself, you understand, for most of it went during the last course of radiotherapy when, with taste buds and throat shot away, I lived on hotel-small portions of Ready-Brek, but the cause of the loss. Somehow it had never occurred to me until a doctor pointed it out the other day that I've lost weight because I have cancer and eating up the pounds is one of the things cancer does.

It means that for the first time in my life I can share jeans with my wife. Ever since I was a teenager I've thought there was something ineffably cool about men sharing clothes with their partners.

I mean, not tights or stilettos, of course, but as a child of tubbiness I always envied those men who would bound out of the college halls in the morning in their girlfriend's Levis.

But that, I'm afraid, is the extent of my new youthfulness. My new little old manliness has nothing to do with age or even of deterioration, but with my own bodily frailty and the state of my bedroom and bathroom and office, all of which are littered with the impedimenta of my new medical routines.

I have little-old-man things I have to do each day with orange rubber bulbs, and special stiff brushes dripping pungent pink cleaning fluids. I have bags full of special foil-wrapped bandages and things made of prosthetic-pink foam rubber which have to be changed regularly. There are tubes I have to change before I eat, and change again after I eat, and which I have to clean with the special stiff brushes and the pink fluid.

Three times a day I potter around the bathroom like a little old man, squeezing bulbs, and cleaning tubes and sluicing parts of my body out and taking pills against pain and swelling and infection and which lie in dozens of bottles piled about the place.

If this goes on much longer I shall adopt a stoop and a little old man's shuffling walk, and put my hand to my ear whenever anyone tries to talk to me, and small boys will shout things at me in the street and I will be mugged on the way to the doctor's surgery.

But it won't go on much longer. I have to hold on to the fact that the chances are that in six weeks the radiotherapy will be over, the hole in my windpipe will be plugged and I'll be eating *Beano*-style mounds of mash with sausages sticking out of them.

Then again, hubris being what it is, I also have to hold on to the alternative, which is that this may be the nearest I will get to being a little old man.

The Times Magazine

20 SEPTEMBER 1997

I AM NOT ME ANYMORE

THE NURSE WHO was greasing up my new tracheostomy tube said that she'd been worried by the depressive tone of the last couple of columns. I laughed as gaily as a tracheostomy allows and said that I have my ups and downs and that if column writing falls on a down day then it could well be that some of that downness might taint an otherwise cheery and upbeat tale of life in the cancerous lane.

The truth is, though, that most of that downness has nothing to do with pain and mortality and everything to do with not yet being able to talk properly. And in not being able to talk, I am not me. Or, at least, not the me I think of when I think of me.

Some of the time I forget that the phrase in my head won't come out of my mouth in the usual way until it's seized up on my lips and the other party has started to stutter apologies for not understanding.

As often, though, I am starting to work within my limitations. I've started gesturing rather than going to the effort of explaining.

Just now Nigella asked me something and I heard myself about to say 'absolutely' in answer, but the word which came out was 'yes'. It's a footling thing, I know, but the John Diamond who says 'yes' is a different person from the one who says 'absolutely'.

Pre-operatively I was profligate with words, throwing away jokes and cracks and little sarcasms to fill up the spaces between thoughts. Now no word is wasted. I use the words I need to use but there is a second busy dialogue playing – but only to me – in the background.

I am talking: talking is what I do. OK, I'm not Oscar Wilde or Moss Hart but to have a riposte or a description or a question sitting there on my lips waiting to be shot into the conversational mêlée and not being able to shoot it is crippling.

And though there are plenty who say that my old incontinency was a bad thing, that it made me facile and unthinking, I enjoyed being the person I was and there are times when I don't enjoy being the person I am. At the back of it all is the most basic question of self-image. Yes, I believe in liking people for themselves, for their pure hearts and their shining inner whatevers, but the truth is that we get on with people because of the way we are with them.

Well, I always have, anyway. I like talky people. Dreadful, I know, but it's how my life has always been.

Thus am I forced to entertain the unwonted thought from time to time: would the people I love love me, know me, have taken trouble with me, if this is how I was when they first met me?

Would my friends, friends in whom I've never had a doubt, have become my friends if, when we first met, I'd been a wounded, honking mute, unable to respond to the simplest question without dribbling?

Would I be with Nigella, come to that? Would I have the kids?

I know I have entered the twitchy land of Jimmy Stewart in *It's a Wonderful Life*, but the answer is almost certainly no.

It has to be: I don't have any friends who are honking dribblers and I am the only honking dribbler among my friends' friends.

Perhaps it should be otherwise, but the fact is that it isn't. It must follow that I am not now the person my friends befriended, my wife married.

I know it's an equation born in late-night depression, that once one starts totting up the what-ifs in a middle-aged life you can get badly, if temporarily hurt.

But I am not me any more. That my friends seem to be

193

willing to do almost anything for me is, I believe in these mad moments, almost worse: they are responding to who I was rather than who I am.

I know that in a month or two, please God, the various therapies will be over and I will be the chattering classes' Mr Facile all over again, but meanwhile this is what disease does to us.

It wrecks our faces and our voices and any talents we may have lying around, and then it makes us separately depressed so that we're unable to deal with the wreckage.

You see? You caught me at a bad time again. Sorry.

The Times Magazine

18 October 1997

THE ODDEST THING

THE ODDEST THING has just happened. I was driving down to the local shopping mall, which multi-million pound edifice is where you have to go hereabouts if you want to buy a 13-amp fuse. I switched the car radio on halfway through that lunchtime slot when Radio Four goes all jocular, and there were a quartet of standard-issue Radio Four panelists solving droll crossword clues for a chuckling Broadcasting House theatre audience.

I could work out who a couple of the panelists were, given how often their voices turn up on the sort of shows where you have to solve crossword clues, or know what Clem Attlee so famously said to Bessie Braddock on Derby Day in 1948, or for two points per ingredient, guess the contents of this medieval recipe for quince syllabub, but I couldn't put a name to the others – even though one seemed vaguely familiar. His was a deepish voice, southern, with a very slight cynical lisp and a . . .

Hold on, though. It was me. It was a programme I recorded, what? Six months ago? Nine? It was recorded in a pre-operative era when I still had all of a tongue and could rent it out for lisping and cynical purposes. Coming unexpectedly upon my pre-cancerous self like that was like looking from the cold station platform into a brightly lit and crowded train and seeing the twin brother I'd forgotten I had idly turning the pages of his paper. Twin, but not identically so, because the other odd thing was the potency of my sense of the me listening being a different me from the me on the radio.

I wrote the other week about the possibility of my being different now from then, and a lot of readers got the stick's wrong end and sent me sweet and encouraging letters to tell me that no, no I'm just the same old me, and maybe I am, because I came home from the mall just as the children came in with Cosima bearing news about some cakes she'd just made, 'made' being demotic three-year-old for having banged the flour sieve around a bit and stuck cherries on top.

I promised here when they were born that I'd never repeat to you the precocious things my children would, I was sure, say, and thus I offer merely as reported speech her assurance that while she understood I couldn't eat the cakes now, she'd make me more when I was better. And it was so cheering to hear, as I always hear from Cosima, the promise of a time when I am well again.

For, knowing no better, she is the only one to discuss my future in the certainty that one exists – no crossed fingers, no litany of please Gods or touch woods, no back-tracking medical qualifiers ending on a rising inflection with '. . . as we all very much hope you will', or, '. . . which I'm pretty sure the blood tests will confirm'.

In fact, Cosima is the only one who so sure-footedly gets the right response to my voice every time. She accepts without second thought the fact that once I spoke like that and now I speak like this, and when she can't understand me she says, 'What?' with none of the apologetic confusion of my friends, who, bless them, can't always decide whether to wait around and hope that a few garbled words will eventually take on meaning within the context of the rest of the garbled sentence, and then realise that these were the key words to my speech and that they'll have to stop me and tell me they didn't understand, by which time they've been pretending to look interested for far too long and . . .

Cosima just says 'What?' though, and says it whatever the context. I'll be telling her off for some infant naughtiness and I'll shout, 'But you know we put the sweets up there precisely so that you wouldn't eat them . . .' and she'll say, 'What?' and manage to maintain the appropriate remorse or fear or truculence all the way through her incomprehension and my repetition, which is some trick.

But not the trick of fifteen-month-old Bruno, who has just got his fifth word, and doesn't realise how odd it is that his father has too. It will be these two who'll get me through, though – Bruno by showing me these things can be learnt and Cosima for showing that it doesn't matter how long it takes.

The Times Magazine

25 OCTOBER 1997

I'LL START WITH THE PEAR

I WAS STANDING at the sink, about to spit a mouthful of baby pear down the waste disposal unit, when I thought, 'No. I shall swallow this pear. I have not eaten a fruit in its true fruitful form since June – the vestigial lemon 'n' lime in the lemon 'n' lime build-up drinks on which I've subsisted for the past couple of months not counting – and I shall eat this one now.'

I almost did, too. And as I almost got it all down my throat, I thought, in one of those tearful moments of mad joy I have from time to time these days, how easy it's all been really.

I'll start with the pear, because that's the quick bit, and then I'll go on to the easy life, because I haven't decided yet whether that's one of the written thoughts that actually goes off for publication.

As you will know, constant reader, they took the back of my tongue out in June, leaving me unable to talk in any meaningful way for a while, although the exact definition of the term 'a while' is still in some dispute. What I wasn't expecting was the effect the new compact tongue – combined, it has to be said, with a second six-week stint of throat-burning radiotherapy – would have on my eating. Who knew the part the tongue played in this sort of thing?

Before I was forced to think about it, I'd always assumed you put food in your mouth, chewed it about a bit, swallowed, moved on to the next morsel. But it turns out that, unless you have a fully functioning tongue shovelling the stuff back towards the gullet as it passes through the scything teeth, the food just stays there at the front of your mouth or, even worse, starts leaking back in the direction of the plate.

Hence the liquidity of my diet these few months past. But it's been two weeks since the radiotherapy stopped and they're talking about taking the tracheotomy tube out of my throat some time soon, and I thought I'd try downing something solid.

So, last night, I started with a pint of Murphy's, which occupies that pleasant intermediate state between liquid and solid and was the first alcohol I've touched since May.

And then I tried some venison stew, of which I managed the part of a single mouthful that didn't fall into the glass of Murphy's as I was trying to gulp it down. That the rest of the stew ended up on the floor was through no fault of my tongue and entirely down to one of the rages I go into from time to time when not being me gets too much to bear.

And so tonight I tried a small, soft pear. Same thing: chew, chew, dribble. The pear was about to go the way of the stew when I thought, 'Damn this thing,' and made it go down my throat. It wasn't exactly Robert the Bruce, but I jumped up and down a little and ran to tell everyone that I'd just eaten a pear.

Which is when I realised two things: that if I was going to eat and talk again, I'd have to make myself do this time after time, day after day; and how, to a large extent, I've lived a life where I've been able to avoid doing most of the things I didn't want to do. Or, rather, wanted to have done but didn't want to do at that particular moment.

I didn't work at school and, true, I didn't achieve what you'd call academic success, but I managed to find a good college where they appreciated certain sorts of academic failure. I didn't work overhard in the job I trained for, but managed to fluke my way into journalism at just the point where I could avoid going through a traditional tedious training full of shorthand and typing. I screwed up a first marriage through indolence, although not that alone, and lucked myself into a second one with the right wife who had the secret of manufacturing perfect kids. Who could have my luck?

And then all this happened – and still I've not been in a position to decide between the easy and the hard hauls: hard as the illness has been, it has been one without choices.

But here I stand at the sink, with strands of pear juice running down my chin, and I know I have to force myself to do this every day until I can do it as easily as you can do it, and for some reason that makes me unreasonably happy.

The Times Magazine

8 NOVEMBER 1997

SORRY, MRS W

MRS RW OF Virginia Water in Surrey writes, 'I am wondering if your illness has anything to do with smoking. Two of my three sons smoke and there isn't a day that I don't worry that they will get cancer of the throat, mouth or lungs. My father died in his mid-fifties of an illness brought on by smoking, so I'm totally paranoid about it.'

Well, what do you think, Mrs W? Of course it's to do with smoking.

Are you listening to this, you two W boys? I smoked from the age of thirteen until some time in my mid-thirties when, a veteran two-pack-a-day man, I swapped the fags for nicotine gum. Or, some days, for nicotine gum and cigars or, on really bad days, nicotine gum, cigars and cigarettes. Has this anything to do with my having cancer of the tongue? I don't want to scare your mother, but she sounds pretty terrified already and so I shall not pull the punch. Ninety per cent of the recipients of my sort of cancer are, or were, smokers. I know, boys, that if you look around you will find people who will tell you that the connection is by no means proved. They will say, Yeah? – well, what about him living on a damned great arterial road with carcinogen-belching lorries screaming through it day and night? Or, never mind, they'll say, the cancer patients who smoke, what about all those contented and steady-handed types who smoke and who don't have cancer, eh? They will tell you about how their old mum smoked forty Coronas a day all her life and died halfway up Scafell Pike on her eighty-third birthday, and about how everyone has to die some time, and you stand as much chance of falling under a bus as you do of catching something nasty from the Marlboro Man.

You will find these people, and if you can't find them you can invent them, and their rationalisations, for yourself. I did, after all, for years.

But two facts remain, lads. One being that this is what can happen when you smoke, the other being that your tearful mother waving this cutting in front of your face won't make the slightest difference. You have probably never met somebody with this illness; I hadn't, either. More to the point, you have met thousands of people with a fag in their hand who look hale enough, who talk without dribbling and eat a meal without coughing it over the tablecloth and don't fix you with a rheumy eye and tell you about the number of tubes an eight-hour operation causes to be poked into you.

I am the walking, talking – or maybe not talking – equivalent of all those schoolday films of blackened lungs and tar-filled test-tubes, the films that never stopped me smoking because the films were about smoking in a different universe – a universe where people got lung cancer and rickety hearts. Everyone I knew smoked; nobody suffered anything worse than weak-mindedness.

Good old-fashioned empiricism tells you that you're safe. As it happens, you're wrong, but there's no way I can convince you of it.

I know this because I know smokers. Smoking friends come round and suddenly disappear for a while and I find them in the garden, the lit fag tucked, like a docker's, into their fist. I say, 'It's OK: you can smoke inside,' and they grin sheepishly at me.

'Sorry,' they say. 'I've cut down. It's just that . . .'

It's as if they expect me to take it personally, as if in some way they believe that I'm insulted by their smoking, by the fact that they can smoke and talk without dribbling and eat without coughing up the part-digested morsels in such an unlovable way. Or, I don't know, perhaps they feel I might think – I don't – that their continuing to smoke betrays a lack of love for me, or they bear some small guilt that the evidence

I present isn't enough to make them give up. But why should it be? The pretend law of averages by which we all work says that my getting cancer reduces their chances of getting it. Who, after all, knows two people with such a rare condition?

So I'm sorry, Mrs W: there really isn't anything I can say to help you as a mother in your fight for your sons' health. But then again, what would you say to help me when I tell you that one of the visitors who nips out into the garden for a quick drag is my mother?

The Times Magazine

22 November 1997

YHJTIOHJOITE

HAVE YOU EVER suffered from sleep deprivation? I don't mean a couple of rough nights when the baby wouldn't settle, or you got back late from a party, but the sort of sleep depri . . .

ZZZZZZZZZ. Wha? What? Who're you? Ah. I see. Right. Sorry. Column. Sleep deprivation, wasn't it? OK. I don't just mean being tired. I mean, you're sitting at the thingy trying to think of the word for the oblong thing in front of the screen with all the buttons with letters on them because at this level you forget the most ordinary words when yhjtiohjoite! Which, apart from the exclamation mark which I stuck in for dramatic effect, is the word you get when a sort of momentary sleep overtakes and your forehead smacks into the oblong thing. It might have been a different word when it actually happened twenty minutes ago: I was re-creating the moment, you understand. In fact I've re-created it a dozen times: sleep deprivation turns you into a two-year-old fascinated by repetition.

Keyboard. Was the word I was thinking of. You see? It's still all there in working order: it's just a bit slow these days. Where was I? Sleep deprivation, forgetfulness, repetition, keyboard . . . Right. Here we go. A couple of months ago when I had the near-death experience which is still referred to locally as John's Near-Death Experience, with all the awe due to its capitalisation, and stopped breathing, they put the blue lights and the siren on, took me round to the hospital and gave me a tracheotomy. Ever since I've had a plastic pipe protruding from just above the top of my breastbone which has to be cleaned and changed a couple of times a week and which, apart from looking pretty grotesque, interferes with such eating and speaking as I'm capable of at the moment.

For the past few weeks, as my scarred throat has started to heal, I've spent most of my waking time with it blocked off with a little red plug, breathing through my mouth and nose as God intended. And then last week I slept through the night with the red plug in and the surgeons determined that the post-operative swelling had receded far enough for me to lose the tube completely.

You can imagine what a panicky prospect that might be considering my last attempt to breathe using my own equipment, but I took comfort in the fact that the half-inch hole in my throat would take a while to heal up. Except it didn't. They whipped it out at midday and by evening the hole had closed itself up to the extent that if I put my fingers up my nose and closed my mouth, I couldn't breathe. No, don't: you would have tried it too.

That was getting on for a week ago and I haven't slept since. Imagine: six nights without any sleep at all. I exaggerate not: I doze off and . . . just . . . as . . . I'm . . . about . . . to . . . ssssleep GRRRKKK I SITBOLTUPRIGHT, WIDEAWAKE as my tongue slips back, my oddly shaped epiglottis – a 'juvenile' epiglottis in the language of ENT people – flops down and I lose my breath.

Sometimes the lack of oxygen causes me to jerk into wakefulness via oddly compact nightmares: tiny little single-act dreams they are, with no plot line and just the one terrifying event to remind me that I'm doing something dangerous. Like trying to breathe.

And so tonight a man is coming round with an oxygen cylinder which counts as good news and bad. The good is that I might get a night's sleep and stop feeling like somebody the army are softening up for work as a grass in Belfast. The bad news is that while losing the tracheotomy was a major step towards looking like a normal person, and eventually talking and eating like one, sleeping with an oxygen tank beside the bed and a set of plastic cannulas connecting it to my nose is somehow profoundly depressing. Only severely ill people sleep with oxygen at hand, or dying ones, and I liked to think that I was moving away from that estate.

For the truth is that with the surgery and the radiotherapy all over, I still don't know whether I'm cured. Nor will I know for weeks, or months, or possibly years. And in the absence of clinical diagnosis, all I have to go on is self-image. Man with an oxygen cylinder isn't quite what I was hoping for.

The Times Magazine

14 MARCH 1998

THE LAST COCKNEY

THE PALL OF Thames fog drifted filthily across the steaming mountains of muck and my friend looked across at me with a supercilious smirk. 'Homesick yet?' he said.

It was meant, in its own minute way, as a joke: as a Chelsea boy he knew well enough that the seething, Dickensian East End we were watching on the screen, the Third World refugee camp of a scavenger community recreated for the BBC's current brilliant adaptation of *Our Mutual Friend*, isn't the East End I mean when I go all nostalgic about the land of my fathers.

But if it was a joke, it was one based, as far as my friend is concerned, on a series of unjoking truths about the real East End as a land of oppressive claustrophobia, of crime and ignorance, of Pearly Kings and knees-up-muvvah-brahn, second-hand cars and dodgy boozers, high-rise diasters and timid gentrification.

His is the media's version of the area and the one which seems to have turned the East End into some sort of home-town metaphor for urban Britain, while maintaining its image as somewhere apart from the rest of the country – a British Basque region if you like. For some time now, the East End has been the area to which otherwise anti-metropolitan pro-gramme-makers have gone if they want a setting in which they can play about with easy local stereotypes, while at the same time hinting that these odd, ill-mannered and dysfunc-tional people are reflections of the rest of us. Or, rather, the rest of you.

It would explain why, having searched around the country for years to find a way of overtaking *Coronation Street*, the BBC found the answer in the gloomy but phenomenally successful *EastEnders* and why, to repay the compliment, ITV has found in *The Bill* a cop-show formula even more successful than the Scouse *Z-Cars*. (They might have guessed *The Bill* would work: *Dixon of Dock Green* had George Dixon fighting polite, small-time East End crime for twenty-one years.)

For we are all East Enders now. It is the natural condition of community Blairism to which attaches our sense of locality, of belonging, of leaving the door on the latch and of joining the darts league. The East End is, like the South Wales valleys and Merseyside, an area to which people claim an allegiance of birth in that irritating Ich bin ein East Ender sort of way, as if the accident of birth gives them – us – special community qualities.

Well, me too. In truth I'm not a complete East Ender: I was born in Stoke Newington which, in those days, was a borough in its own right and one with a north London postcode at that. And although Stoke Newington was later subsumed into the entirely eastern borough of Hackney, I'm not sure that a birthright can be retrospective. Whatever: I grew up in parts of London with E postcodes – in Shadwell, Stepney and Hackney. For the couple of years we moved out to Essex in my infancy it was to Debden, an overspill estate full of families from Shadwell, Stepney and Hackney. It was the move detailed in *Family and Kinship in East London*, the work of urban anthropology which gave the local intelligentsia their mythic status before Pinter and Wesker were around to do the job properly.

I lived in Hackney until I was sixteen, returned there after I left college, taught there for a few years, left, eventually, when I was thirty-nine and remarried a woman who, with a sense of the right and wrong side of the Park, made moving westwards effectively a condition of betrothal. If anyone knows, I should know what an East Ender is.

But I don't.

I have a New York-born friend called Reggie Nadelson who, for much of the year, lives in London, where she writes rather good detective thrillers. She decided to set part of her next work in the East End. Could I, she asked me, jot down a few notes on what an East Ender actually is, where he lives, what it is which divides him from the dreadful north Londoners or, worse, the grunting savages south of the river who cluster around Danny Baker for warmth.

I tried. I started in Stepney, which is where my great-grand-parents lived when they arrived in Britain, as did my grand-parents and parents after them. But the Jewish East End isn't there any more: it's moved out to the lusher suburbs of north London and the residents only ever see the old homelands when they dash in, pressing the central locking system as they cross the North Circular, for emergency supplies of bagels from Brick Lane and Ridley Road.

In its place is Bengali East End, but there wasn't much I could tell Reggie about that. A few years ago I stayed for six weeks or so in my brother's flat in the centre of the area, sur-rounded by street signs the names of which I'd first heard in stories of family mythology forty years earlier: Flower and Dean Walk, Tenter Ground, Old Montague Street. The kosher butchers were halal butchers now, the synagogues had had minarets added to them and become mosques, the broken-backed Jewish men who shuffled along Brick Lane had been transformed into broken-backed, shuffling Bengali men.

With the impenetrable language and tinkling music, the pungent-smelling food and the odd clothing, it all felt worry-ingly alien to me. Precisely as alien, I imagine, as my lot had seemed to the indigenous population then. Or, at least, a pop-ulation which had achieved indigenity for, like all dockside areas, two generations settled in the same place counts as a long-established family, and in the old dockside villages of Limehouse and Rotherhithe there are still Swedish chemists, Norwegian churches, Chinese restaurants run by descendants of the people to whom Conan Doyle sent Sherlock Holmes to score his opium.

Who else could I tell her about? The dockers? Men who made their living from the smallness of the world but whose imaginations rarely extended beyond the parish boundary, men whose lives were run by the union, who passed their jobs from father to son, whose own traditions maintained a strict demarcation between them and other East Enders? Except that there are no dockers now: the East End is no longer a place of arrival and departure.

The dockers have gone because the docks have gone, to be replaced by Conran restaurants and warehouse apartments and the headquarters buildings of franchised niche-marketing operations and, yes, newspapers like this one. Most of the local industry has gone with it – either because it's moved to where the docks are, or out of London, or because it's done what British industry has had a disturbing tendency to do over the past couple of decades.

What remains is nothing like the East End I remember from my childhood, and nothing like the East End of Dickens. My Hackney is, as it always was, a slightly run-down inner-city district, no different, once its glamorous riverside neighbour has lost its *raison d'être*, from Moss Side or St Paul's. Parts of the borough have been gentrified in a hopeful sort of way by chancers who imagine that if they paint the front of their houses to look like Georgian Islington or Hampstead, they will acquire a status based on something other than the history of geography.

And the rest of the East End, the Alf Garnett docklands backwoods of West Ham and Plaistow, or Poplar, where a voting ward is named 'Lansbury' after the socialist leader, or Canning Town and Beckton and the ribbon-developed wastelands leading out to the Ford works at Dagenham? Without the docks and the Isle of Dogs, they are as anonymous as the inner-city hinterlands of any medium-great city.

So when Reggie writes her book, what will make the East End special? Possibly its new anonymity – always useful in a thriller – which even Dickens might have understood. It means that I'm probably the last generation who will be able to boast of being an East Ender, or who will want to. But happily, it will also mean the end of that maudlin boastfulness by those simpleton historians who believe things were better when the East End was still famous for its crime, and death and slums.

The Times Magazine

18 April 1998

IN THE NAME OF SCIENCE

Pass me the reins, will you, ostler? Today I feel like riding my highest horse. The other week there was one of those let-the-public speak TV programmes in which a man was given half an hour to put forward an argument which, the programme publicity announced, 'challenges conventional wisdom'.

This programme was made by a man who performed experiments on animals and aimed to show that, within generally agreed limits, performing experiments on animals was a reasonable way of going about things. Infuriating, isn't it? How, in this day and age, can people believe such things? Can it really be the case that there are now so few people who believe in the righteousness of animal experimentation that it counts as 'unconventional wisdom'?

When I was a schoolboy there was a general consensus between the anti-vivisectionists and the scientific establishment that some six million animals were killed in the name of science each year. That was as far as consensus got: the antis talked as if most of the six million – and what an evocative number that is – were tortured monkeys; the mad scientists would point out that 90 per cent of the experiments were on anaesthetised and unphotogenic rats and mice.

Nowadays the consensus is that there are just three million or so animal experiments, but to listen to the antis you'd imagine that represented an inexorable climb rather than a drop by one half.

The reason I'm on a higher horse than usual about this is because I've just about reached the point where, had I not been operated on last July and irradiated in the subsequent months, I'd be dead. It could have happened, of course: I could have taken the advice of those who told me that various plant extracts would do the job just as well, or that all radio-therapy cures were lucky spontaneous remissions masquerading as science.

But I didn't, and here I am. And one of the reasons I'm here still is because of animal experiments. Animals were used to test the mechanical and physical efficacy of the radiotherapy machines, to perfect the intricate surgical procedures which have been developed over the years, to test the various drugs which have kept me breathing and mainly pain-free. We can argue, if you like, about whether there was an alternative to animal experiments and whether scientists could have got away with using clean and cheap computer simulations rather than messy and expensive animals. But the fact is that animals are what they used, and animals seem to have done the job. I could have been dead, but thanks, in part, to a large number of dead rats and a few dead dogs and rabbits I'm alive.

Again we can argue about the morality of this. You can tell me that if it were you or your child or spouse or parent you would take death rather than accept any medical procedure which had been tested on animals, and I will believe you. But when I go to the hospital I see hundreds of people who are willing to undergo those procedures knowing full well the animal connection. And in other waiting rooms, surgeries and chemist's shops around the country are millions who know the same thing.

They know it for the most part because we all know it nowadays, but also because the anti-medical mob try to make sure we know it. As it happens, I'd like to see the medical community making a bit more of the help they get from animals rather than leaving it to the anti-medicals to do the job, but I'd guess that a survey taken in my hospital's crowded waiting room would show that 90 per cent or more of the patients knew that animals were used to improve on cancer treatment.

Pro-experimentation isn't, as the BBC seem to believe, 'against conventional wisdom'; it is conventional wisdom.

What has happened is that the broadcasters have started to believe there is a proportionate connection between the amount of fuss made about a thing and public support for that thing.

There. I have ridden my high horse humanely, gently, without letting it break into a sweat. But if it became necessary to kill the horse to save my life or that of my human loved ones, I'd be there like a shot.

The Times Magazine

25 April 1998

THE HARD SELL

THE SELF-STYLED car supermarket a couple of miles away has become a sort of local theme park, and on fine Sundays whole families turn up with their car price guide under one arm and the Thermos under the other, looking for the car they might one day, but not usually this day, want to buy.

There are thousands of cars there, all waiting for new homes, and the dads stroll up and down the rows, pressing their noses against each driver's window, shielding their eyes with their hand so that they may better read the car's mileage and divine whatever it is they think they can divine from mileage.

The sons run from car to car, trying the locked doors until they find one which a salesman has left open. The wives, for the most part, spend their afternoon steering husbands away from the impossible Mercs and the Beemers and towards the cheap Rovers and Fords.

I have been that father. Not with the Thermos, I grant you, and usually on my own, but I've been to the reception centre – decked out in carpet tiles and catalogue office seating like a Third World airport – and I've asked for the keys of a nearly new Jag, and I've sat in the leather front seat trying to force the repayments into making some kind of economic sense.

And then the other day I went for real and, chicken that I am, finished up looking over a Saab of the same rank and colour as my current one, but with fewer years under its Swedish belt.

A salesman strolled out into the drizzle with me to show me around.

'It's a Saab 9000,' he said.

'Yes,' I said, 'I know. That's what I asked to see.'

'Right,' he said. 'Right. So you know the car then?' He said this as if I was trying to do him out of a job. What's the point of having car salesmen if the punters already know the bloody cars?

I looked over the machine, trying to remember the things you're meant to do to second-hand cars. I prodded a couple of rubber belts and held up the dipstick, as if the oil running from it might coagulate into a word or two of help: 'rusty nearside wing' or 'knackered big end'. But it just looked like oil.

'Can I have a test drive then?' The salesman looked at me, trying to gauge whether a man with my voice was likely to have a driving licence. 'Are you going to buy it then?' 'What do you mean?' 'If I let you have a test drive, are you going to buy the car?' 'I don't know. That's why I want the test drive.'

'Yes, but if I let you have the test drive and the car drives OK, will you buy it then?' 'You mean I have to agree to buy it before you let me have a drive?' He looked nervously towards the main office. Perhaps, he seemed to be thinking, I was a pretend customer sent out by the directors to test him.

'It's the company rules. I have to ask you, otherwise I can't let you have a test drive. Are you going to buy the car?' He wanted me to lie. He wanted me, I knew, to say, 'Yes, I'll buy it' – even though he knew I didn't mean it – just so that he could stop asking the ludicrous question over and over again.

'But it's not just the test drive, is it?' I said. 'It's all sorts of things. I mean, I'm not certain I want to stay with Saab.'

Actually, this was a lie. I'm not given to product placement in this column, but a few years ago a London bus drove into my side door at some speed when it skipped a light, and I walked from the written-off car entirely unscratched.

'Any other car, you'd have been dead,' said the policeman who came to breathalyse me and the bus driver. I'm sure there are other cars which save lives, but this was the one which saved mine.

The salesman stared at me hard. Was I being wilfully stupid? Just say, 'Yes.'

So I said, 'Yes.'

And, just to spite him, I bought the car. I got home and I said to Nigella, 'I've just bought a car,' and she gave me the look wives give husbands when they've gone out to buy cars without prior consultation, and she said, 'What was it? The hard sell?' And I said, quite honestly, 'I don't know.'

The Times Magazine

20 March 1998

WINDSOR? NAH, *WINEBERG*

I AM TURNING into my late great-aunt Kenia. I have many fond memories of Auntie Kenny. The most vivid is of her and her sister Etta sitting in front of my grandmother's TV scrutinising each programme's credit roll for Jews.

'Warren Mitchell,' she'd say as the actors on *Till Death Us Do Part* were credited and add, meaningfully, 'Warren *Meisel*, as was, of course.' Or 'Bernard Bresslaw: Brady boy' because, as far as much of my family was concerned, every London Jew was branded for life by the East End youth club he or she'd attended long decades earlier. And a Brady boy was as different from an Oxford and St George's boy or a Stamford Hill boy as a Brahmin from an Untouchable.

Other relatives were less discriminating. 'Bruce Forsyth!' Aunt Fedya would cry as that entirely Gentile entertainer's name appeared on the screen.

'No!' Uncle Simmy would say. 'Bruce Forsyth? Brucie? Really?'

'Certainly,' Fedya would say. 'Forsyth? Ha! Finkel! You know the Finkels used to run that bakery on Hessel Street?' and she'd give a look.

It wasn't just the stars, either. I've sat with her as she watched the list of craft and technical workers scroll up the screen.

'Lerner . . . Goldman . . . Frankel . . . look! A Cohen! Robinson . . . Levin.'

'Robinson?'

'*Rubenstein*,' she'd say as if it was the most obvious thing in the world that the chief electrician on *The Adventures of Robin Hood* or the make-up supervisor on *Z-Cars* was a Jew with an anglicised name.

There were members of my family who knew the secret Jewish provenance of every member of Equity, every journalist, every rock singer, every sporting hero – including my grandmother, who used to refer to Norman Cowans, the black cricketer, as Cohen.

My grandfather had the same trick but on a global basis. His membership of some vital Board of Deputies sub-committee charged him with counting all the Jews in the world, as if he were some sort of Jewish Hercules – 'And, Alf, when you've finished that, I want you should go down to the Negev with a teaspoon . . .'

For a long period of my childhood, we'd turn up on a Friday night and the first thing he'd say on opening the door was, 'Guess how many Jews there are in Nepal?' We'd say we didn't know, and he'd say, 'Go on, guess.' We'd say, 'Five,' or '100,000,' and he'd say, 'No – seventy-four' in an excited voice as though about to give us their names.

Anyway, I've started doing it.

The giveaway isn't that I sit in front of the box and say to my wife, 'Goldstein,' when the name comes up, but that I have accepted the shorthand which my family always used. Nobody ever says *why* the names are being called out, or what they represent, either as a commentary on the TV business or on the assimilation of Jews.

And, in truth, I haven't yet got the affliction quite as badly as some of my family. So far, I've only found myself shouting out names when there's a particular irony – as in the BBC's sitcom, *The Vicar of Dibley*, where, by my reckoning, there are at least three Jews on the parish council.

It's reasonable enough that a group of people which has been chased around the world in various nasty ways should take some pride when some of its number get their names in lights. I certainly understand why Jews of my grandparents' generation who had experienced the chase at first-hand *shepped naches* with such glee.

But it occurred to me the other night, as I was pointing out

218

that three-quarters of the production team of an American film about Christmas had names ending in '-stein', that there's another group which takes the same pleasure.

As I mentioned last week, any journalist who mentions his Judaism in the British press is immediately put on the mailing list of some of the shady groups operating from box numbers in south London. Every so often, one such group will send out a booklet modestly entitled: *The Threat to Civilisation!* or *Mothers Beware!* detailing the Jewish takeover of Britain's culture or economy.

These booklets are no more than long lists of Jews divided into occupations; a sort of Jewish *Yellow Pages* without the phone numbers. The last one I was sent listed all the Jews in the media and show business, and I realised that it wasn't just my family – and possibly yours – sitting in front of the TV and listing the names of Jews; the anti-Semites are doing *exactly the same thing*.

I imagine they're doing it in a different tone of voice, but you take my point. What's more, they seem to be doing it with about the same level of accuracy as my aunt Fedya. Their latest effort is full of men and women who are not only *not* Jewish but who never were.

It's hardly surprising, though. I was once sent one of these booklets from an outfit in Ireland. It was rather better printed than the average piece of hate-mail, complete with fuzzy photographs, essential to the author's belief that you can tell Jews from the way they look.

Among them were photos of Prince Charles and Princess Anne: two Britons whose easily obtainable family tree goes back to Pagan times and doesn't include, as far as I understand it, any Jews. But no, said the author, 'We have no definite proof that the Royal Family is Jewish, but if you look at their faces . . .'

Shame, really. If only they'd get their lists a bit more accurate, they could at last serve some useful function – a checklist for all the Aunt Kennies of this world. Wouldn't they be pleased?

Jewish Chronicle

29 MAY 1998

OY, IS THIS LANGUAGE COURSE

A PAIN!

I HAVE TO tell you that all this is wreaking havoc with my spell-checker.

You know about spell-checkers, of course: little gadgets attached to word-processing program which make a computerish tutting sound when they see words like, well, computerish and tutting, as it happens, neither of which words are in my computer's dictionary and both of which appear on my screen as I write with a wiggly red line underneath them to show that the computer wants to know whether those are really the words I want to use or am I just winding it up again.

Normally, I am careful to pass my writing in front of the spell-checker: I have an irrational horror of my work turning up at newspapers and the sub-editors rolling on the floor screaming: 'Look! The idiot spells "embarrass" with one "r".'

But, over my weeks in this space, the computer has started noticing words it's never seen before, strange, alien words which start with a guttural *ch* and go downwards from there.

Worse: they are words which I know I have spelt wrongly because I have written them one way and seen them in print in another. There are, I know, at Furnival Street, sub-editors who roll on the floor, clutching their sides and screaming: 'Now he thinks you spell "gutkas" with an "ers"!'

My parents, ever sensitive to their firstborn's embarrassments, solved the problem with a birthday copy of *The Dictionary of Popular Yiddish Words, Phrases and Proverbs*, written by one Fred Kogos and published in, of all places, Secaucus, New Jersey. To it, they added the current hot seller from the Educational Services Corporation of Washington, DC, in their top thirty language tapes: *Yiddish – Start Speaking Today!*

It takes a while before the teach-yourself-Yiddish tape starts putting individual words together in sentences, but once novices have got used to counting to 1,000, and how to say hello and goodbye, the tape moves straight on to the useful stuff:

'*Ikh fil zikh nisht gut.*' (I don't feel well.)

'*Vos iz mit dir?*' (What's wrong with you?)

'*Di fis tuen mir vey.*' (My feet hurt.)

You can see how the language defines a whole culture, can't you? I bet in *Teach Yourself Italian*, the first faltering sentences after the basics are: 'Want to come back to my place then?' and, in French, it's something useful to do with snails; but, in Yiddish, it's: 'My feet hurt.'

One rather feels the tape should do the job properly, though, and instruct learners how to join those three words so that they mean: 'What d'you mean, how do I feel? A lot you care. My feet hurt, since you ask, but you'll forget I told you because I already told you yesterday and already you've forgotten. Not that your feet wouldn't hurt if you had had the life I had. It's not just the feet either. Did I tell you what the doctor said about my back?'

Let us move to the next exchange, remembering that these are the phrases you will need to learn, according to our tutors at the Educational Service Corp, before you learn how to order a meal or what eating utensils are called:

'*Mayne eltern zaynen nisht gezunt.*' (My parents aren't well.)

'*Vos iz mit zey?*' (What's wrong with them?)

'*Zey hobn hertsveytik fun di kinder.*' (They have no heartaches from their children.) Their children, no doubt, who are writing sarky pieces about their birthday presents.

Before it moves on, the tape stops to instruct us to one final *kvetch*: '*Vos iz mit dir?*' (What's wrong with you?) '*Di beyner tut mir vey.*' (My bones hurt.)

Now, I've checked with some other phrase books; in other languages, you learn how to say you've cut yourself, or have a stomach ache or a broken limb. It is only in Yiddish that you are expected to complain that your *bones* hurt.

Note that magnificent plural: we are not talking about a bruise or a knock but about that vague malaise where suddenly all your bones hurt and you can't go to the kalooki night or do the washing up.

But, if the tapes give us the Yiddish speaker as *kvetcher*, the book has him as something surlier. In a section entitled, 'Instant Yiddish – Jewish Words and Key Phrases to Help You Get Along Anywhere in the World', we don't have a chance to complain that our feet hurt because our first task is to look for a hotel.

I've been trying to think of parts of 'Anywhere in the World' where you would routinely walk up to strangers and ask them for directions *in Yiddish* but, apart from small areas of Jerusalem, Brooklyn and Montreal, I can't.

Nonetheless, I shall give Fred Kogos the benefit of the doubt. We are in Beijing and we need a hotel, so we get out our Instant Yiddish and: '*Vu iz a guter hotel?*' (Where is a good hotel?) It goes without saying that, in Yiddish, there seem to be no words for 'mediocre hotel', let alone 'youth hostel'. Yiddish-speakers expect only the best.

Indeed, as soon as we're shown the room: '*Es gefelt mir nit.*' (I don't like it.)

The book doesn't actually say, but I get the impression that Fred Kogos thinks you should say this as a matter of routine, just in case they think you're some *shlemiel* with hurting bones who will take any old room so long as he can get his sore feet into hot water.

'*Veist mir an ander tsimmer.*' (Show me another room.)

At last, we're settled in the second room, we've ordered breakfast (*bulkes un kavel*) for seven a.m. (*zaiger in der fri*) and we're ready to see Beijing. We ask the porter for directions to the important tourist sites. And what is the first site we ask to see?

'*Zogt mir, zeit azoy gut, vu iz doh an apteik?*' (Tell me, please, where is there a drug store?)

You can see it now: the couple back from their retirement trip around the world, the two of them in their comfortable shoes looking nostalgically through their photo album: 'Do you remember the romantic place in Rome where you bought the aspirin and they gave you a free crepe bandage?'

'Of course. And look: here's the little *shopke* in Paris where that man looked into my eyes and told me I was beautiful and then sold me that stuff that cleared up my gas problem in two days flat.'

'Magic moments, darling. And just think: it's all because we spoke Yiddish.'

Jewish Chronicle

5 September 1998

THE PROBLEM WITH CANCER

I'LL TELL YOU the problem with cancer. I don't mean the problem, which is that it kills 60 per cent of the people it touches, but the day-to-day problem for the likes of me. The problem is that it doesn't feel like cancer.

Almost every other illness, disease, physiological disturbance or anatomical failing comes with its own set of symptoms. You have a runny nose, a splitting headache and a dry throat and you know that you have a cold, or, if you're a man, flu. One collection of pains and wheezes means bronchitis, a slightly different collection means pneumonia, a different collection again means emphysema. The symptoms give a diagnosis and once you've had the diagnosis, you can relate the symptoms back again to the disease you know you have. Eat a chicken vindaloo, feel the pain, say to yourself, 'Ah yes: that must be the peptic ulcer the doctor mentioned.'

But not cancer. Or not my form of cancer.

I have developed some interesting new symptoms, most of which are so basic that were I to describe them to you you'd certainly say, 'Poor sod: he must have some sort of mouth cancer,' which in fact is usually what I say to myself. Every so often I collect up any new symptoms I have and take them along to my surgeon, who puts me in a sort of upright barber's chair and sits opposite me with his legs spread around mine and my knees touching his inner thigh. It's the only way he can get close enough to look inside my mouth and it's the most intimate thing I've ever done with another man since I stopped playing rugby, and yet even though we've sat together like this dozens of times, neither of us mentions the intimacy.

Sometimes he'll search around with a dental mirror and a spatula, and sometimes he'll go the whole hog – or as much of the hog as is possible in a Harley Street office – and put a fibre-optic tube with a tiny camera lens at its end into my nostril and down through my various cavities until it reaches the area where the symptom seems to be. Once in a while he'll send me back to the Marsden with a chit for a CT scan or an X-ray, just to make sure, but thus far there seems to have been a rational explanation for each new symptom, an explanation which doesn't involve cancer, but does involve the recovery from its treatment.

Whenever I do go back to the hospital for one of these non-invasive tests, he waves me off with a sanguine see-you-in-a-month-or-so farewell as if both he and I know that the test is a complete waste of time given all the other cancerous criteria which I don't fulfil, and as often as not he spoils the effect by phoning me with the results in a voice full of relief, saying, 'Great news!', as if the idea that I might last out the month has come as a complete surprise.

This time we've gone a stage further and tomorrow I go into hospital carrying pyjamas and a toothbrush. He will put me under and search around to check on the current symptoms with a touch more rigour than he can bring to the wakeful throat.

And this is, as I say, the problem. I have these symptoms which could be the symptoms of a recurrent cancer and then again could be the symptoms produced by a set of medical coincidences, which I regard as unlikely – but then what do I know?

Because unlike the cold or the hernia or the thyroid condition, there is no set of symptoms which feels incontrovertibly like oral cancer. Indeed when you read about the symptoms for most cancers they always seem to be ones you might mistake for something else. In most other circumstances I might have some inner sense of whether I have the illness or not, but not with cancer. I go through the days sometimes convinced that it can only be the worst and then an hour later the only

225

thing that reminds me that I was just preparing to die is the slight soreness at my jaw where I was clenching my teeth.

All of which is why I won't be in this space next week. I can't even ask you to wish me luck because given the exigencies of magazine publishing it will all be settled by the time you read this. Wish it me anyway, though, will you?

The Times Magazine

12 September 1998

FIFTY-KILO SACK OF FLOUR

I GOT A letter the other day from a baker. It wasn't even so much of a letter: more a short note. He'd read, he said, about my being ill. He had cancer too. One day he'd been fine, working away at the mixer and the ovens, and now here he was a couple of weeks later dying. The thing was, he said, that at least I could write, whereas he couldn't even lift a fifty kilo sack of flour any more.

He'd underlined 'fifty kilo sack of flour', but there was no more blunt recrimination than that: I can carry on doing that which – as far as he can see – defines me, but he can't even do that simple hefting job that he's taken for granted for all these years. I'm not sure what he wanted from me – for me to stop writing, to get worse, to understand that I was relatively lucky – and, unsure of the legitimate response, I was going to write back and say that just as I'm more than a writing machine, so is he more than part of the bread-making apparatus, and not to worry, but I never did. There comes a point where cheery advice just sounds fatuous.

And anyway: his implication is right. It is unfair. It's unfair for him, and for me, and for the leukaemic child and for the eighty-four-year-old who's got through a good life but wants another decade. It's unfair for our wives and husbands and children and friends. And, against all the odds and despite all we know, we still expect things to be fair.

But the stakes might be levelling between the baker and me because it turns out that the cancer is back. Or, more likely, has been here all the time. And although I suppose I've known for weeks or even months that I was due this news sometime soon, actually getting it changes things. I don't just mean changes things in terms of expectations, although there's that too, but changes the way I feel about myself.

My perpetual languor is, I now realise, not that of somebody still recovering from a lengthy operation a year ago ('You'd be amazed how long it can take . . .') but of somebody whose strength is being sapped by the multiplying cells. And the pain isn't, after all, the pain of a cut and sutured tongue trying to find its old mobility but of the ulcerated and granulated flesh tugging at the nerves.

So here's what happens. Last time they cut away about a third of my tongue and pulled the two cut ends together. This time most of the other two-thirds goes. They replace it with a lump of skin-covered muscle taken from my back which will form some sort of mass in my mouth against which I can bounce words.

If the transplant takes particularly well then I might even be able to speak better than I can at the moment, because one of the things that happened when they discovered I still had cancer was that the mobility of my tongue wasn't up to much after all. For months now, sundry therapists and surgeons have been telling me that one of the ways they could tell I was making a reasonable recovery was that my tongue was becoming mobile again; now it turns out that not only was it not becoming mobile, but that this was, all along, a warning sign.

There is good news, though, which is that this is still the old cancer rather than a new one popping up at arm's length from it, and that if the surgeons slash and burn in the right way then I have a reasonable chance of a cure.

Meanwhile, by the time you read this, and if things go well, I shall be in the High Dependency Unit, which is what they call intensive care nowadays, breathing and feeding and peeing through various tubes, living on a diet of liquid gunk and morphine. It won't be fun, and it's not fair, and I'm particularly angry that I won't be around to see my daughter in her new school uniform when she starts school this week, and while I won't be in this space for a while, at least there's an evens chance that I'll still be able to lift fifty kilos in a year's time, which is, I now know, a blessing to be counted.

The Times Magazine

228

3 OCTOBER 1998

THROUGH THE MIRROR

FUELLED BY THE morphine, which turns dreaming's scatter-gun impressionism into neat and formal narrative, I must have had the Miraculously, His Voice Returns! dream half a dozen times over the past fortnight. It comes in various versions linking various parts of my life – voice returns in the staffroom of the school I used to teach in, voice returns at the magazine I worked for fifteen years ago, voice returns at a party the summer before last – which makes it, I suppose, rather like drowning incredibly slowly and your life running before your eyes in a stop-frame motion.

Normally I wake up just as I break the news to a happily weeping family, but a recent version went on to the end: the sudden rediscovery of my vocal powers, the slight and not unattractive lisp which is all that remains of the surgery and the return in triumph to the microphone.

Which is odd, because knowing, as I now know, that I won't broadcast again is the least of it. I was only ever a print journalist talking his writing into the mike or the camera, and it is only as a fatherly story-teller, husbandly joke-maker, chatterer to friends, scorner of enemies, that I miss the voice. Or miss its prospect, at least, for as things stand I'm not sure what it might be that I will have instead of a voice in six months' or a year's time. Last time I was here I know I said that there was a chance that the operation would actually improve my voice, but that turned out to be as probable as Shergar coming back to win the next Grand National.

You will know that I have an almost childish belief in the

229

power of modern medicine, and therefore when I speak of its failings it's not because I'm one of those modern cynics trying to find some reason in the randomness of physical nastiness by forever giving the latest smug statistic of the amount the medical profession doesn't know. But there is some part of me which feels that I've fallen foul of some medical con trick. I'm not saying that I think that I've been tricked out of the tongue and the sundry other glottal accoutrements which the surgeons have just spent some time and skill whipping away, for I'd have lost those anyway and, by the scalpels of less-skilled surgeons, more besides. Rather, it was the creeping but unseen inevitability of it all, the swiftness with which black turned to white and I was through the mirror and into a new world.

Every so often since the big operation last year I would visit my surgeon, who would look inside my mouth, ask me some questions and tell me how well I seemed to be doing. Without carving me up every week such a pronouncement could only ever be made on a more-or-less clinical basis, but generally speaking it seemed that all those symptoms which I took along to my surgeon's rooms were signs of improvement. Those pains were nerves knitting; that food trap was a perfectly normal sinus growth. Moreover, my bruised tongue was starting to get some movement back, my voice was improving and my nights were ever more restful.

Until the other week, as I reported here, I had a full biopsy and suddenly those very same details became symptoms not of improvement but of recurrent cancer. The pains were tumour growth, the food trap was a sinus in the tumour, the lack of movement in my tongue was obviously suspicious and it was apparent that my voice wasn't improving as it might. And strangely all these pronouncements were made as if they were the logical continuation of the opposite pronouncements made the week before. The shepherd who had one night looked at the red sky and told what delights it augured looked the next morning at the same red sky and pointed out that it was that very redness which was the warning.

Either way round, here we are again: half a step forward and twenty back. The surgical word is that this time they've done for the bastard and that now all I have to do is learn to live with an unclear future. Will I ever eat again? (At the moment I suck in liquid food through a tube in my stomach.) Will I ever talk in words that anyone other than Nigella, the children and speech therapists can begin to understand?

For those readers who were looking forward, but certainly no more than was I, to the column returning to its former jollities, I'm afraid that I can offer no more than this: now read on.

The Times Magazine

17 October 1998

MY FIRST OFFICIAL SWALLOW

IT'S RIDICULOUS HOW grateful one becomes for the tiniest achievements. I went for my first official swallow last week. Since the operation, not a morsel has passed through my gullet, for while they were relieving me of a tongue, they also stripped me of the various sub-glottal flaps and folds which make sure that food goes to the stomach and air to the lungs. You have epiglottis, false vocal cords and, as a last – literal – gasp, the vocal cords themselves to stop food going down the wrong way. I have only vocal cords, and I've had to spend a couple of weeks learning how to close them while swallowing a sip of water.

There are some in my position who will simply never swallow anything again and for whom the stomach tube is their chum for life. The good news, I hope, is that my surgeon is a resourceful sort of chap and has managed to rearrange my windpipe, larynx and sundry other bits and pieces so that liquids of the right constituency and amount hit the entrance to the oesophagus before they get to the trachea.

That at least is the theory, but when you're moving bloody and swollen bits of interior furnishing around through a hole made in the neck, it's not always easy to know where everything will be when the bleeding stops and the swelling goes down, hence my banishment from swallowing until I was passed fit to do so by a committee of surgeons, speech therapists, X-ray technicians and the rest.

To tell the truth, I thought I'd fail. With the tracheostomy in, I have the weakest sort of swallow and when the odd toothpaste rinse slips over into my throat, I tend to spend the next half-hour coughing away unmerrily. But in front of half a dozen experts of the swallowing committee, I stripped to the waist and stood in front of an X-ray machine pointed at my throat and connected to a TV camera and videotape.

They switched the X-ray on and the extent of the interior carnage was immediately apparent. Although from the outside I look rather better than I have for the past decade or so, an X-ray cross-section showed the gaps where the organs weren't, the new diversions taken by various items of plumbing, the missing back molars where the surgeons needed to make space – and somewhere in there, a pair of meagre and insubstantial vocal cords, leaving a massive tract waiting for the liquid to pass into my lungs.

Lisa, the speech therapist, prepared a tablespoonful of lemon-smelling ('flavoured', I have to take on trust) liquid and went through the routine again. Deep breath, bear down 'as if constipated', sip, swallow, cough.

I took the sip of cold liquid and felt it pass over the parched drop at the back of my mouth, into my throat – and down into my stomach. On the X-ray I could see the swallow: the oesophagus clenching, the vocal cords closing, the tiniest drip spilling over into my windpipe and being coughed back on track again.

I grinned as if I was personally responsible for this series of entirely involuntary contractions and tiny acts of gravitational force.

We tried it again, this time with a slightly thickened mixture. Straight down, no messing. 'Cough,' said Lisa. 'You must cough.' I was getting cocky: I made a notional 'ahem' sound and grinned again. We tried it with yoghurt, with a soupy mixture, with some more water: I swallowed the lot.

And then I found myself weeping. In six months of teetering backwards towards the abyss, it was the first time I felt myself going forwards. Suddenly there were all sorts of possibilities. I may not be able to fully engage in a family dinner, but I may one day be able to do the soup and the custard and, come to that, the wine and the port. I could do more than just swill iced water round my mouth in the hot weather, and suddenly my beach fantasy became realisable. I'd forgotten about it until then, but as I was being wheeled from my room into the theatre four weeks ago, I asked Nigella to describe the four of us on some sunny beach in a year's time: it was an image I wanted to hold with me as I went under.

As I swallowed the last small gulp and they turned the X-ray machine off, that was what I remembered again.

Of course, one swallow does not make an autumn, and I've never done quite as well since as I did in the hospital that day. But it will come back to me, I know it will. And I will be the one slowly gulping beer on a beach next year.

The Times Magazine

7 November 1998

HOW TO SLEEP

I'VE FORGOTTEN HOW to sleep.

I don't mean I've become an insomniac, simply that I've forgotten how to do the little trick you do that gets you from waking to sleeping. Worse: it suddenly seems such an unlikely thing to be able to do. Lying there, awake, thinking, sentient, hearing the rumble of the District line down the road and of the passing lorries, seeing the little red lights on the TV and the stereo, feeling the bumps in the bed and having an involuntary conversation with yourself about the price of a new mattress, and then – click – out of it: deaf, mute, blind and generally senseless.

How do you do that? Why would you want to or need to? How do you turn off all the sensors that evolution has given you, ignore the creaks and twitters and partnerly snores, and sleep?

No, don't tell me: I've tried it.

For a couple of weeks after the operation it wasn't a problem: the combination of the sort of painkillers that point out that if affected you shouldn't drive or use machinery the next day plus a sleeping pill kept me pretty sedated most of the time, as you may have noticed in my writing. But when I came off the other drugs I found the sleeping pill (or, more accurately, sleeping juice: it has to be able to go in the feeding tube) let me sleep between about midnight and three in the morning and then forced me to go and write unreadable chapters of a novel until dawn.

One surgeon suggested booze, and so I pumped four glasses

of what the label said was a rather good red into the tube and saw it appear again a couple of hours later as a thick and undistinguishable rosé.

Relaxation techniques? Tell me about them. I learnt a guaranteed routine by which each part of your body gets heavier and heavier, weighed down by unseen forces, heavier, heavier, heavier – except by the time I get round to the left forearm the right knee has forgotten to be heavy and is all light and twitchy again and can feel the agonising weight of the duvet and every crease in the sheets. I've tried reading bad books and reading the sort of good books that are meant to send one to sleep. I've tried staying up late and going to bed early, sleeping with more pillows and with fewer.

Nothing works.

And so I lie there thinking. Or, at least, not quite thinking but sort of being but with the occasional thought. The crypto-thoughts aren't particularly deep – the other night I found myself deciding which cleaning products I'd need to bring up from the cupboard in the basement if I wanted to make a really good job of the bathroom – but they get me from hour to hour. You'd be amazed how many hours there are in a night: every so often I look at my watch and find that it's only two or four or five, and I'm never sure whether I want it to be earlier so that I stand a chance of sleeping before morning or later so that I can get up and hope the creeping tiredness will stay with me through the day and into the next night so that I may sleep.

Up to a point it does: the days crawl by in a fug of doziness and then at midnight I'm wide awake again. Or, rather, I'm as dozy as ever but without the first idea of how to translate that doziness into sleep. There are, apparently, people who spend a lifetime like this, and others in strange Third World countries who use it as a form of torture. But for me, for the past couple of weeks, it's become just another slight worry somewhere in the middle of a list of a couple of dozen worries. Perversely, the greater worry is that I keep on finding myself worrying whether the daytime tiredness is a sign of some recalcitrant cancer hiding about the place.

I think, though, that I have found some sort of answer, and

that is gin. 60cc of gin mixed with tonic and a lemon-flavoured vitamin elixir I use, pumped up the tube just before bed, stays where it's put and does the world of good. It doesn't send me to sleep, but then again I don't mind so much about being awake.

The Times Magazine

11 December 1998

THE FUNNIEST THING SINCE
STEVE COOGAN

ON A PARTICULARLY arid Friday night (can you believe that Bruce Forsyth is, in this day and age, given a full half-hour of prime time in most regions to play *Bruce's Price Is Right*?) let me offer a word, if I may, on behalf of Sacha Baron-Cohen. I've never met the man, have seen him only rarely and briefly on television and all I know about him is that he's not long down from Cambridge, but for my money he's the funniest thing since Steve Coogan put on his Pringle V-neck and became Alan Partridge. Baron-Cohen's speciality is funny voices, an affectation I can usually do without, but he does voices nobody else has ever considered doing.

For a while, he appeared on the Paramount Comedy Channel as the camp presenter of a fictitious Austrian fashion programme who would turn up at the catwalks of Milan and Paris interviewing self-obsessed designers at purposeful cross-purposes. On Channel 4 recently he turned up as a finger-popping hip-hop interviewer pitched against pillars of the establishment who had been led to believe he was the real thing. The former Judge Pickles on the subject of 'when murder is, like, legal' will, I hope, ensure that he gets even less punditry work than he currently receives. Tonight, Baron-Cohen appears on *Comedy Nation* as Christo, the Albanian reporter, and it's worth sitting through the rest of the programme just to catch him.

Sunday Telegraph Magazine

19 JUNE 1999

THE MEAL THING

THERE IS A particular sort of burger you get only if you order it through room service at the ritzier type of American hotel – if, of course, ritzy can be used as a generic description of hotels which aren't themselves the Ritz. It is sent up under a silver cover on a flat plate the size of a Mini Cooper tyre and is a cordon-bleu impression of what an ambitious cheeseburger might be like given a better start in life. It is invariably served juicily rare and bloody, comes with thick wedges of fresh tomato and onion and, in a sort of post-modernist joke, is accompanied by teensy miniatures of Heinz ketchup and Tabasco sauce.

It's a meal I've had perhaps a couple of dozen times in my life, but for some reason it's the meal I think of when people ask what it is I miss most about not being able to eat.

That and Toffee Crisp Clusters. Not that I've ever tasted a Toffee Crisp Cluster because they've only been on the market for a matter of months, but every time I see the advert for them I think: that could have been me there eating that Toffee Crisp Cluster and now I'll never know what they taste like.

I can have a guess, of course, having lived with taste-buds and a functioning tongue through the long years pre-Cluster, when the Toffee Crisp came only in bar form (indeed, I can even remember the giddy years of the too-short ascendancy of the Coffee Crisp in, I think, the Sixties), but I will never know whether the taste experience works, as it were, in miniature. You think I exaggerate for literary effect but, I promise you, I wouldn't bother throwing such exaggerations around for such nugatory results. I do genuinely feel aggrieved, albeit momentarily, when the ad comes on.

The same goes for the new custard snack that Birds have brought out, with a little tub of yellow cornflour paste attached to another little tub of biscuit fingers. There's hardly a chance I would have bought one had Messrs Birds conceived the neat idea of flogging custard by the centilitre before my tongue pegged out, but still the missed chance rankles. The world of snacks is moving on and leaving me behind. It's hard to believe, I know, but I have never tasted a Nestlé Wonka, and never will.

The result is that although I was strictly meat and two veg in my previous life, I have become something of a food obsessive. I find myself wandering downstairs purposefully just when Nigella and her assistant, Hettie, are in their most vigorous Fanny Cradock modes and pulling hot and reeking pies and puddings out of the oven like magicians pulling flags-of-all-nations out of their pockets. I watch, most days, things like *Ready Steady Cook* on afternoon TV, and am able momentarily to imagine that I could recreate the dishes for myself. I read cookery books and the recipe sections of magazines and papers, and the other day I so completely forgot that I am past eating that I chucked a round, hard chocolate into my mouth, and then had to do a headstand to stop it choking me.

Worse, I dream about food. Not long after the operation I started having the occasional dream in which, fully glottal, I would eat a whole meal and, of course, discuss it with everyone around the table. My subconscious, though, seems to have got used to the idea that I don't do the eating thing any more, and so now I have dreams in which I have lost my tongue and am unable to eat all but one specific food. The other night, for instance, I dreamt that I could eat only doughnuts, and last night the dream had me eating a rather specific orange-flavoured pudding from the island of Menorca, although, as far as I know, no such pudding exists.

Oddly, I have speech difficulties in these dreams, too, but I somehow manage to overcome them in such a way that my almost complete lack of speech becomes merely a rather attractive impediment. I suppose I should resent these impossible dreams as much as I do the late coming of the Toffee Crisp Clusters, or the custard pots, but there are nights when I find myself pumping in the odd sleeping elixir and actively look forward to a comatose meal rather as teenage boys look forward to erotic dreams for lack of the real thing.

The Times Magazine

31 JULY 1999

THE MOST UNLIKELY

OF EXPERIENCES

OVER THE PAST couple of years I suppose I must have turned up at the hospital to hear bad news, what? Two dozen times? A score? Whatever, the point is that based on the prognoses given to me on previous visits I've never arrived expecting to hear the worst. Each time the news that I have cancer, that it's spread, that it will involve this operation or that procedure and will result in one or other new disability, has come as something of a surprise. Each time I have taken the doctors at their word when they have told me that my chances were excellent, and then good, and then mediocre, that this was probably the last operation I'd need, that I'd be back to my old normal self in a month or two, or six.

Not this time, though. It's not that I'm any more cynical of their prognoses, you understand, merely that we've reached the end of the list of possible positive results.

The chemotherapy is finished, although it's taking me some time to get over it, and I still don't wake before lunchtime most days. Or what would be lunchtime were I still of the lunching orders. And so last Friday I went for the scan which would determine whether the chemo had worked or not. The results wouldn't be available until the following Monday, and so the two of us spent the weekend in various forms of nervous denial, what with a dinner at the Ivy, a restaurant not too grand to provide me with an un-menued broth which I could syringe into my tube, and chatty afternoons getting drunk among the kids in friends' gardens.

And when Monday came I realised I was about to undertake

that most unlikely of experiences: I would walk into a room where a man would tell me how long I had to live.

I imagine that believers of fortune-telling shuffle into Gipsy Petulengro's tent with the same sort of apprehension, or they might if any fortune-teller ever predicted anything other than a long life. (In fact, not long before the cancer was first diagnosed, I wrote a piece for one of the women's magazines in which I compared the fortunes offered to me by half a dozen professional seers, from end-of-the-pier crystal-ball readers to computerised astrologers to high-society tarot merchants. Not one of them predicted the cancer or anything less than the full three score and whatever it is nowadays.) For the first time I knew before I turned up that there would be no suggestion that the result of a test might be that I was cured or free of the cancer and the hospital place which goes with it. The only options would be that the chemo hadn't worked, in which case I would have X months to live, or that it had and that I had Y months. Z months, where Z equals the restoration of a normal lifespan, is no longer an option.

We sat reading old magazines in the waiting room, and eventually Lynda, a research nurse who maintains precisely the right, calming balance of professional decorum and chatty fondness, came past and said that while the doctors would have to give us the results, we shouldn't worry. Five minutes later we were called to see my oncologist and my surgeon, who gave us the good news which is that the chemo seems to have worked and that I'm in remission.

I didn't realise until I got outside, dizzy and sweating, the extent to which I'd been holding my breath while I waited for this news, while at the same time blocking out any real thought about what it means. And the bizarre thing, even more bizarre than going to see the man who will tell you how long you will live, is that I found myself joining in with the conspiracy to believe that this is good news. Good news would be that the cancer has gone away for ever.

The Times Magazine

27 November 1999

ON DEATH ROW

Somebody said the other day that it must be like being on death row, being me. The comparison is closer than they can know. The sentence has been delivered, and every so often a call comes through from the state governor's office postponing the date of execution, but never in such terms that I'm allowed to believe that one day the sentence itself might be commuted to something less irreversible.

Yesterday, for instance, I was shaving, and found myself prodding the operated-on and mangled bit of my neck where the razor will never quite do its job. Was it my imagination or had it started swelling slightly?

I took a census round the house – Nigella, Nigella's assistant Hettie, our au pair Lisa. They looked, and furrowed their brows, and said they thought so, maybe possibly, they wouldn't have noticed it if I hadn't pointed it out, but now I came to mention it . . .

Nigella phoned Peter Rhys Evans, still, after all these years, the surgeon with his name on my cancer. He booked me into his clinic at the Marsden the next morning and a small team of people inspected me in the way that cancer surgeons do, the set of their faces constrained by not knowing quite what news they might have to deliver.

And gradually, as the inspection grew more complicated, I got more worried. I'd gone in to be reassured that I was just being paranoid, that there was no swelling at all, that I was imagining it all. But by the time I'd been palpated and then scanned, and then ultra-sounded, I realised they were taking it seriously, each level of inspection announcing that the previous level hadn't been conclusive.

In the end they stuck a needle into the swelling and sucked out some cells for examination. What, I asked the doctor, was his hunch? He made that doctor's face again and said that although the scan hadn't shown anything definite, the ultrasound had been a little more suspect and he wouldn't have taken the cell sample if there hadn't been a possibility of, well . . . Nowadays I come across a lot of sentences which end in three dots. He gave it fifty–fifty.

We got home and a friend popped round. We told her about our morning. Oh yes, she said, she'd noticed the swelling last week, but hadn't thought to say anything.

Over the two-and-a-half years since this started, I've spent some time being scared, but never have I been quite so sick-in-the-stomach terrified as between the moment he made his fifty–fifty pronouncement and the time thirty hours later, and an hour or so before I write this, that he phoned through with the results, which were negative. Or, rather, not positive, which shade of meaning is slightly different and is a back-covering way of saying that although there was nothing cancerous in the sample they took, who knows what may be elsewhere.

I was certain that they'd find the cancer had come back. And, of course, I was told when the chemotherapy started that if – or, rather, when – it did come back, then that would be it. I've spent the past thirty hours doing my usual obsessive's routine of playing patience on the computer ('If I win one of the next five games then it'll be negative. OK then: the five games after that . . .') and going over with Nigella the conversations we had with the various doctors to try and divine extra shades of meaning from their attempts to speak neutrally. Nigella, for instance, in a moment of pessimistic insight, thought that when one doctor said, 'We haven't seen you since July,' what he might have meant was, 'We never promised you more than remission, did we?' And I've been going heavy on the poignancy-of-life business. I keep on finding myself staring at objects around the house and trying to work out whether we acquired them before or after the first

245

diagnosis. 'When we bought that chair', I hear myself saying, 'I had no thought of cancer,' or, 'The day we got that picture framed, I was living an entirely different life.' I can still remember with ridiculous clarity, given the mundanity of the event, the act of choosing the chair, of deciding to frame that particular picture, but not what it felt like for cancer to be something which happened to other people, of not waiting for the governor to ring through to the jail and say that there are no more reprieves.

The Times Magazine

5 February 2000

IT'S THE ONE ABOUT . . .

I TRIED TO tell a joke the other day. It's the one about the little boy who finds a pair of welder's goggles on a rubbish tip, and the dodgy geezer who turns up in a beaten-up Jag and offers him a ride, and if you don't know it, I'm sorry but it's not suitable even for a page this far back in a family magazine. We were sitting in the pub, all telling jokes, and I started to write this one down on paper, and after one line Toby said: 'It's the one about the welder's goggles, yes?' So I told him to tell it, in the hope that we could get it over with quickly and I'd get the laugh as the original donor of the joke, but he went into one of those 'OK: there was this man. No, sorry. This boy, right? Is that right, John? . . .' routines. You know the sort of thing. Eventually, between us, we crawled on bleeding knees to the punchline, which got a polite titter but no more than that, and I realised that joke-telling was another trick I can't do any more.

It was an odd week to make the discovery because this was the week I found a new joke-telling voice. A producer friend at the BBC asked me to write her some sketches for one of those late-night sketch shows on Radio Four. I've written a few hundred radio scripts in the past, some of them containing the work of a jobbing banterist, but I've never actually written anything which starts 'FX: pub atmos – enter MAN 1 slamming door', and which has a proper punchline. Not that punchlines are compulsory in these post-*Python*, *Fast Show* days, but I'm an old-fashioned sort of sketch-writer, it turns out, and I feel uncomfortable if there isn't a collapse of stout party at the arse-end of a sketch.

They used a couple of the sketches and asked for some more, which pleased me no end, but not as much as the discovery the next day that I still seem to have a voice.

I met a teacher on the Internet last year when she was still a trainee teacher, and although we'd never met in person we agreed – I'm not sure how – that it might be useful if I came into her school and lectured her twelve-year-old girls on smoking and the perils thereof. It makes sense, after all. When teachers talk about smoking, what they say is that if you do it you'll die, which is meant to be a serious threat but really isn't because a) most people have seen lots of smokers but have never seen one clutch his throat and fall over dead, and b) because from a pretty early age we get used to the idea that we will all die, and dying from smoking seems as reasonably unlikely a way as any other to go.

What's more, the other lesson that most people are given about smoking is that it's terribly addictive, which is true enough, but looks ridiculous from the point of view of a non-addict, who can't possibly imagine what addiction to something as mundane as nicotine-enriched smoke might feel like. The idea, then, was that I go in and demonstrate that before you die of smoking you go through something which is worse than a quick and painless death, and that such is the addictive quality of the weed that even people in my position still use it.

The lecture went marvellously. The girls asked preternaturally bright questions (although one put her hand up and asked timidly if they could see the tattoo) and gasped at the right moments when I showed them the various scars, and I think I might do some more school lectures from time to time.

But what was most encouraging was that after about ten minutes I gave up using the overhead projector to talk with and started using what passes for my voice. I don't know whether it was because I was standing up, or because there was precisely the right configuration of phlegm and saliva and uvula that morning, but they seemed to be able to understand every word I said.

To celebrate I went out and drank rather a lot so that nobody could understand what I wrote, let alone what I said, but at least it made up for not being able to tell jokes any more.

The Times Magazine

6 AUGUST 2000

WHAT IT'S LIKE TO BE YOUNG
IN GLASGOW

EXTRACTS FROM THE first few minutes of *Tinsel Town*, mostly declaimed in various shades of Glaswegian and all set to a soundtrack of high-energy-techno-garage-hip-hop-rave-a-pop-a-doodle-doo, or whatever that music is that sounds like a very loud, very scared fly trapped in a bottle.

Young boxer in training swings punch: 'He's takin' the *pess*!'

Boy in school uniform comes through front door, rushes up stairs, throws himself on bed, beams joyously as fly-in-bottle music comes over Walkman headset.

Young undertaker looks baleful and longs for weekend.

Young woman thrashes young man on PlayStation while smoking joint. 'I'm dumping Ian tonight.'

Two young coppers can't be arsed to nick young car thief because it means filling in forms.

Young man irons trousers in sitting room preparatory to going out.

Young man demonstrates sensitivity by a) listening to talk radio rather than fly-in-bottle music, b) emptying mother's hidden booze bottles down sink.

'Why not just dump him?'

'We're going to have a great night tonight. Remember those uppers I got?'

'I really thought we had something . . .'

God, but I'm glad I'm not young, aren't you? Perhaps you are young, of course, but there will come a day when you're glad you're not and that day will be when you watch a television series aimed at the young and you're so relieved you don't have to watch the second episode.

And trust me: that day will come, because eventually *all* series will be aimed at the young. Alan Titchmarsh will be replaced by a bloke called Gaz or Jez or Boz in shorts and bleached hair who'll makeover people's gardens by planting rows of cannabis; the news will be read by a woman called Nikki or Vikki in a Versace T-shirt who can't quite remember who John Major was, or why; *Panorama* will reveal the scandal that is the door policy on inner-city dance clubs; and *Going for a Song* will be introduced by Gail Porter, who'll ask the teams to guess how much this Britney Spears combination hip flask-condom box is worth.

For everyone in television is obsessed by getting a young audience. The average age of the cast of *EastEnders* has dropped, by my estimation, by around fifteen years since the series started all those years ago. *The Bill* is, I'm told, about to lose another lot of its more mature characters and is now referred to by some of the cast as *Grange Bill*. Even *Neighbours*, once a bad soap opera about a group of Australian suburbanites, is now a bad soap opera about a group of Australian suburban schoolchildren.

Why this obsession with the young? Because commercial stations believe that the young have money which they'll spend on advertiser's products and the BBC believes it has to do everything ITV does to keep its ratings.

Of course, this may just be me being middle-aged and sour and rehearsing the televisual equivalent of how fresh-faced all the coppers are now – except that whenever I speak to a middle-aged television producer or manager they crease their already creased foreheads and tell me how hard they're striving for a young audience and have I got any ideas for a sort of *Family Fortunes*-type show that could be presented by an alternative comedian for twenty-five-year-olds? Which is why we have series like *Tinsel Town*. Don't get me wrong: it is beautifully shot and directed, but that's about all. Being for young people, no shot lasts for more than ten seconds and no scene for more than thirty. It is the dramatic equivalent of a pop video, where the premise is that you don't have to take in dramatic events, chunks of dialogue or plot details as long as you walk away with a vague impression of what happened. It's television to watch while stoned or after a couple of alco-pops. 'Love, drugs and clubbing in a city [Glasgow] that lives for the weekend,' as the BBC describes *Tinsel Town* are, I suppose, valid subjects for drama, but I'm not sure what the point is of simply trying to replicate the sensations of love, drugs and clubbing on the small screen. It's as if the second series of *Walking with Dinosaurs* consisted of no more than the sounds of rustling leaves with the occasional loud roar as a diplodocus hoves into view. Certainly that would give us some idea of what it might be like to share the earth with dinosaurs, but that's all it would give us.

All *Tinsel Town* gives us is the sensation of what it's like to be young in Glasgow. My guess is that if you're young, you'll prefer the real thing, and if you're not, then you won't much care either way.

Sunday Telegraph Magazine

26 August 2000

DUMB SUICIDAL BASTARD

GOD, BUT I hate smoking. It's all the standard stuff, of course: the smell – or, worse, the fact that now I don't even notice the smell the next day – the ash everywhere, the wheezing, the knowledge that a fag in my hand is the equivalent of having 'dumb suicidal bastard' tattooed on my forehead, well, you know the litany. If you don't smoke you know it because you quote it at smokers and repeat it to me in e-mailed sentences starting, 'However, I was disappointed to learn . . .', and if you do smoke, you know it better still. I love smoking, too, of course, for reasons I can't, or needn't explain to you, but partly because I know enough about myself to understand that if it wasn't cigarettes it would be something else – booze, cocaine, jogging.

But as a victim of smoking I have extra reasons to hate it. Not because of what it's done to me, although there's that too, of course, but because my starting again seems to have turned me into a walking totem for so many other idiots.

There are the wood-knockers, for instance. These are the fellow smokers who see me light up, holding a finger to my tracheostomy tube so that I can get vacuum enough to draw, and give me a verbal equivalent of a slap on the back. Good ol' Diamond: smoking to the last. What a character, eh? Want a light, John? Try one of these, John: no filter and extra tar siphoned in at the factory. No, hold on to the pack, really: I've got two more in my pocket.

I'm in Italy as I write, staying as the guest of a friend who insists that the legend '*Nuoce gravemente alla salute*' printed on

Italian fag packets means 'Your government salutes you' and is a thank you for buying from the state-owned tobacco monopoly, and about half of us here smoke. Bright, intelligent, creative people, all of us, and all dumb as hell. But pleased as I am to get letters from readers who say that my descriptions here helped them give up, I also know that those around me who smoke take some comfort from seeing me with a cigarette at my surgically twisted lip. Like a nicotinic Jesus figure I am suffering so that they may not: I'm the one who got unlucky and while they're around me, and while I'm still around, they will escape.

But worse than them are the non-smoking libertarians. You know the sort: the ones who believe in the God-given right of Philip Morris and British American Tobacco to preach the word that tobacco is a life-enhancer, sexual stimulant, social mixer, because we have an equally valid right to say no. I hate them twice over: once because of their smugness; the second time because of their gracelessness. They are smug because what they are saying is that clever old they have passed through an obstacle course which has tripped up stupid old us. The libertarian creed is one held by those who believe only themselves to be capable of the smart choice in any given situation. People who are ill, or skint or addicted are in that state entirely because they are stupid and the more free some of us are to be stupid, so the more free are the libertarians to demonstrate their own smug good sense.

But they are so graceless in their smugness. We go to stay for the weekend with libertarians – non-smokers who have ashtrays on every side table as proof of their libertarian tolerance of their fellow man's right to kill himself. I light up. They smile, thinly. I blow out the smoke. They move backwards. I move my hand slightly; an ashtray is placed within flicking distance in a way that suggests anyone sufficiently proletarian to have a cigarette is equally likely to grind out the stub on the Axminster when he's done. They come into a room in which I've been smoking and give a stage-covert sniff as one might in somebody else's dubious lavatory. The ashtrays aren't there for ash, but as a political symbol, rather as a very ex-student activist might keep a bust of Mao on the mantelpiece next to the flashy dinner-party invitations.

253

Don't get me wrong: I understand why they might not like me lighting up in their houses, why they might not like the smell and the smoke and the ash. I just wish they'd say so, send me to smoke at the end of the garden, confiscate the fags at the door, rather than pretending to collude in an act of libertarianism in which they – and I – really don't believe.

The Times Magazine

23 SEPTEMBER 2000

THE LITTLE THINGS

AND THEN THERE are the little things – the things you would never guess could come about when you hear the diagnosis. It was at the height of the petrol blockade about ten days ago or so. Empty roads, full buses, everyone whistling 'Pack Up Your Troubles in Your Old Kitbag' and telling each other that it'll be over by Christmas. Imagine, then, how smug I was that I get about on a Vespa with its hundred miles to the gallon. (Yes, I know the last time I talked two-wheels to you, it was the Harley. But it was nicked, as Harleys are born to be; and I discovered that zipping round London on a scooter as some sort of ur-mod was more fun than togging up in leathers every time I want to post a letter.) Except that eventually even the Vespa ran out of petrol. No problem. The Land-Rover was sitting in front of the house with a couple of gallons left in the tank – fuel enough to get a Discovery up the road to Sainsbury's, and possibly not back again, but plenty to get a Vespa home to the factory in Italy. I found some rubber tubing, stuck it into the Discovery's tank, and started sucking. And then stopped. With a tracheostomy tube still hanging out of my neck, my sucking power isn't up to siphoning petrol. And, naturally enough, the idea of half a gallon of premium unleaded going into my lungs didn't appeal.

I popped round to the local car parts shop for a siphon. They were, of course, out of them. So was the next shop and the one after that, and if I'd gone any further there was a substantial danger that I'd run out of the little petrol I did have.

So, I went into Mothercare and asked for a breast-milk

pump. I mean, is that lateral thinking or what? Edward de Bono, eat your heart out. 'What do you want a breast pump for?' said the woman behind the counter, which, as questions go, is even more bizarre than my asking for the thing in the first place. Why would she think I'd want it for anything other than pumping breasts? And even if she did, what of it? I started to write on my pad, 'My wife has just . . .' and she said, 'You want it for petrol, don't you?' I nodded, as if this was some sort of shameful admission. 'Well, we're out of them.' I don't know why she was so fierce about it. Perhaps there had been a run on breast pumps and she was worried about evil motorists having a good time at the expense of genuine nursing mothers.

Boots sold me one, though. It took me a while to convert the thing from milk to petrol. Handy DIY tip: cut the last quarter inch off the nipple and use insulating tape to get rid of the air leak around the breast pad. Eventually I got it to move half a pint of water from the sink to the kitchen floor, and I was ready to try it with petrol.

I stuck the rubber tube in the petrol tank and started pumping. And pumping. And pumping. Nothing. Which, as far as I remember, is just what happened last time we tried using a breast pump. I pulled the tube out and detached it from the pump, leaving the rubber breast plate exposed. I put my hand over it and pumped to see whether I could feel any suction, but it turns out the hand is wrongly conformed for a pump designed to fit breasts and I couldn't get a good seal. I tried it on my cheek, but these days my cheek is too sunken for good suction. And so I lifted my T-shirt and – well, I put the thing to my breast. And pumped.

Which is why the policeman, who was passing at just that moment, saw a man with a tube through his neck standing in front of a Land-Rover apparently trying to pump milk from his own breast.

He started to ask me what I was doing, but somehow didn't seem to be able to frame the question. I smiled winningly, with that smile that says, 'Yes, I know this looks odd, officer, but I promise you there's a reasonable explanation,' while at the same time drawing my free hand across my throat in that

'I don't have a voice' motion that I do. He gave a nervous grin back, and walked on. I suppose he was thinking of the paper-work that would result.

How the story will play in the station canteen, I really have no idea.

The Times Magazine

21 OCTOBER 2000

THE ALTO SAX

AND SO WE continue our fascinating journey through John's lymphatic system, and in today's episode we'll be watching the cancer cells as they take up residence in that most traditional of all their homes: the lung. Or, possibly, near it: until I have the bronchoscopy in a couple of days' time we won't know just what the eerie shadows on the scan really mean.

'I suppose there's no chance that it's benign, is there?' I asked Dr Shah, the lung specialist who, post-scan, has been added to my medical retinue. He raised an eyebrow and pointed at that X-ray of the slice of lung which most graphically illustrated the problem. My problem. 'I wouldn't have thought so. Would you?' he asked as if we were discussing a dodgy universal joint on an old Cortina.

The bronchoscopy involves scraping off a bit of whatever the shadow is to see whether it's a good cancer or a bad cancer. Who would have thought there was a choice? They're relative descriptions, of course. As far as I can work out, 'good' means it's the same flavour as the cancer I already have and thus may be battered into some sort of remission by more radiotherapy. Bad means they hold off on whatever treatment they can think up until the time when, as Dr Shah put it, I need it most. I guess – and I was beyond asking too many questions by this time – that means that we're talking palliative care only.

The strange thing is that I haven't had any real symptoms of this. Not until the diagnosis, anyway. 'Can you climb a flight of stairs?' asked Dr Shah. Well, yes. No problem. 'Two flights?' Of course. We have two flights at home. I run up them most times. 'What about three flights?' I paused. Who knows? Why would anyone want to climb three flights of stairs?

The thing is, though, that when doctors start asking me questions to which the answers might indicate serious problems, I always think that the answer I give might actually affect the problem – that if I say I can run up eight flights of stairs while smoking three Woodbine untipped then I shall show myself to be healthier than the scan demonstrates me to be and thus, in some mad way, become healthier.

Perhaps I should have told Dr Shah about the saxophone, too. I've played the alto sax for years now – well, I say play: I do the saxophonic equivalent of Chopsticks, picking out old pop numbers note by note from books which promise they can make me Charlie Parker by next Thursday. Except that I stopped playing two or three years ago when after some medical excursion or another I found myself too weak to blow the thing. And then last weekend we went round to my parents and I picked up Dad's clarinet and without thinking tootled a verse and chorus of 'I'm Beginning to See the Light'. I came home and found – what do you know? – that I could do the same on the sax, and so I've started playing again.

So I came back from the hospital numb but, as I thought, symptomless and started playing 'Someone to Watch Over Me', which seemed suitably mournful, and watched as, prompted by Ellington's notes, a largish clot of blood eased its way out between the flange in my tracheostomy tube and my chest. I coughed into a handkerchief: more blood. Look! A real cancer symptom of the very sort which sends people scurrying to the doctor saying, 'I think I may have cancer.' But then again, between scan and diagnosis I may have been cured. Or, I should say, healed.

I recorded my annual appearance on the Ruby Wax talk show the other night, this year with a computer keyboard rather than the illegible notebook I used last year. I was on with a healer. You know about me and healers, don't you? Exactly. And I started off giving him the full sceptic treatment, replaying to his every claim with 'No you haven't' or

'No you can't' or 'No you didn't.' But what can I tell you? The claims he made seemed to be marginal to say the least, and he seemed as sceptical of them as anyone at the table. I liked him. I let him press the back of my neck on camera. Hell: I asked him to do it. I may be a sceptic, but when you're sitting next to a bloke who says he's killed off cancer cells in the laboratory, it would be foolish not to let him have a quick rub.

And who knows? It might have worked. Actually, I know: it won't have.

The Times Magazine

8 DECEMBER 2000

TWAS THE WEEK BEFORE YOU
KNOW WHEN

Twas the week before Christmas and all round the shul,
Sprawled the marketing team of Kvetch, Cohen, O'Toole.
(That's Avrom O'Toole, a true West Hendon boy,
but whose father's great-gran was a Donegal goy.)
Old Man Cohen stood up and, his cheek fiery red,
Turned his good eye (the left one) on his colleagues
   and said:
'It's months since this project upon us was wished
So far we've got nowhere, got nothing – *gornisht*!
It's not like it's really a difficult thing
To make Chanucah go with a Christmastide swing.'

From his seat at the back rose young Isidore Kvetch,
The son of the founder, a tall, well-dressed wretch,
And, op'ning a folder, proceeded to run
Through the focus-group findings for NW1.
'The problem, it seems, is somewhat iconic,
A matter of symbols, of signs – it's ironic,
For what I am hearing from ABC1s
Is the *goyim* have got all the marketing guns.
They've got Santa and Rudolf and tasty mince pies,
Saints Joseph and Mary, Saints Morecambe and Wise.
Herod, Harrods and Deb'nams and Boxing Day sales
And poems (like this one), nativity tales.
There's the Queen's Christmas message and the babe in its
   cradle.
And what have we got? Just some oil and a *dreidl*.'

The three men fell silent, for what could they say?
They were up against something much greater than, er,
   they.
'Tradition,' wailed Cohen, like some squat, new-age Tevye
Bemoaning his fate to his partners, his *chevrah*.
'We had it for ages. It worked so well for us
Now it's theirs, and they're rich, and we're not – just out
   tsores.'

It was Abie O'Toole's turn, and he paused ere he spoke;
Then he said: 'I believe I'm an ordin'ry bloke,
All I want in this season is what every man wants
Just my kids round the table, paper hat on my bonce,
Some food in my belly, a glass full of booze.
Maccabi or Jesus? Well, any excuse.
But think, lads, just think – when was Christmas invented?
Not the tale of the infant and his parents, prevented
From finding a room in the inn or a house,
But the *modern-day* Christmas, all THAT *mishegas*.
It's all the concoction of Queen Vic and her hubby,
A German called Albert, sort of bearded and chubby.
He sold her the package, all that pine trees and snow.
And holly and ivy and – well, I don't know.

'But, boys, if we're pushing the Chanucah deal,
It's not poor Joe Public who should hear our *spiel*.
We must go to the top, where real power is.
To her highness, her greatness, her *goyness* – Queen Liz!
Sell *her* on the *dreidl*, the oil and the light
And the next thing you know – "Des's Chanucah Night"
With Gaby and Jamie and Wogan, *begorrah*!
All fighting to turn on the West End *menorah*!

'With her on our side, it'll just run and run,
There'll be "Chanucah Special" on BBC1
With Brucie and Jimmy both doing their *shtik*,
And *EastEnders latkes* on sale in the Vic.
And *dreidls* on *Countdown* and kreplach on *Corrie*
(The Rovers could take on a barman called Morrie).

And Radio Four? How far down can they dumb us?
It's a new panel game – hey! – *What's My Shammus?*
We'll kosher the Archers and all of their ilk
No more they'll farm barley, just honey and milk
With Phil Archer a *frummer* – look, Cohen, don't knock it,
And up at the cowshed a new, live-in *shochet*.

'The shops will fill up with new Chanucah toys,
With Finchley Road Barbie and – one for the boys –
Action Man in his *kipah*, and his miniature Uzi
And his female sidekick – little Six-Day-War Susie.'

And that's how it happened – except just for this:
The Queen wouldn't buy it. 'No way,' said our Liz.
'I'll do Jewish High Days – a *Pesach*, a *Succos* –
But hyping up this? You can *kish mir im toches*!'

Jewish Chronicle

31 December 2000

REASONS TO BE CHEERFUL

Like most journalists I'm loath to let light in on the magic that is the editorial process, but this was the first commission I've had in twenty-odd years in the game which read quite so much like an extract from a suicide note. 'Just tell me, John, what the hell is the point of it all?' said the e-mail from the editor, although it probably had somewhat more potency before I coyly changed the word to 'hell'.

Bizarrely, people hint at much the same question all the time, although few of them put it quite so starkly or are prepared to pay me to try and answer it. This is hardly a boast: were you in my position, they might do the same to you. They think I know something nobody else knows, that I've found the secret answer to a question which, through fear or embarrassment, they can't quite bring themselves to ask.

My position is this: I have an apparently terminal disease which doesn't allow me to make any realistic plans for more than a couple of months ahead, a voice which stopped when my cancerous tongue was removed, a diet entirely dependent on the food blender, and a fair to middling amount of pain on most days. To add insult to cancerous injury, I neither feel the need of nor can I discover any comfort in religious faith and I take refuge, legally or otherwise, in no more than the occasional dose of mind-nudging drugs.

And yet most of the time, and within the usual limits, I seem to be happy, even – given my willingness to accept commissions like this one – smugly so. What, they want to know, is the trick?

Well, yes, there's the nice house and the reasonable income from a cushy job that lets me show off in public the loving wife and family, the circle of supportive friends who indulge me in my various whims. To that extent, I suppose I have it all, or as much of it as it's possible to have under the circumstances. But those circumstances do make a difference: I might have it better than most tongueless terminal cases, but I know of no scale against which one can compare friends, family and possessions with the prospect of a long and healthy life. Would I swap a child or a friend or the family house for a new working tongue and a clear scan? Don't even ask, and not least because I'll never have to make the choice.

But it's a fair assumption on the part of my inquisitors: with so little time left for living, what is there to live for?

The easy answer is Philip Larkin's about none of us ever being able to get out of bed in the morning if we had any real sense of our own mortality, and it seems to be an answer borne out by the mortality statistics. Depressed and fraught as we're all meant to be with our fast and unlivable modern lives, last year only 5,000 or so of us were so desperately unable to cope with it all that we killed ourselves, which ranks the act of suicide alongside one or two of the less common cancers as a cause of death. Even if we don't know what there is to live for, we all want to carry on living. Well, of course we do – it's what we're programmed for. A species which could take life or leave it alone wouldn't get anywhere like this far in the lottery of evolution; I imagine that death is as much of an unwanted shock to the day-old and senile mayfly as it is to the average Briton who has reached the age at which death is to be expected.

Indeed, before all this happened to me I used sometimes to wonder what it must feel like to be seventy-eight or eighty-two or ninety and wake up every morning knowing not that today might be your last, but that whatever happened the chances were against life continuing for much longer. How, I wondered, could the Saga company sell holidays to all those elderly types in their elastic-waisted trousers and their treble-E fitting sandals? What were the customers expecting to bring back from their gentle cruise in the Med? Memories? But surely they have enough memories. What can you do with memories when you have only months or a few years to play with them? How can you relax on that cruise when every morning you wake up surprised still to be here and anxious that tomorrow you might not?

Except that here I am, a nominal forty-seven but in the position of an energetic and slightly breathless ninety-year-old with most, but not all, of his faculties, knowing that the chances are against my seeing more than one more birthday and yet I wake up as keen as ever I was to improve the shining hour. I am as happy as I seem to be, yes, but that's because this side of sociopathy or advanced religious zealotry we can only take so much happiness before we are saturated with it. We have a limited capacity for happiness, but an almost infinitely unlimited capacity for, well, not unhappiness exactly, but non-happiness.

Which, I imagine, is why much of the time we are as fulfilled by the various forms of personal non-happiness – anger, disappointment, envy, hatred, frustration, fear, alienation – as we are by contentment. This article, for instance, is a rarity in the British press, with its chirpy positivism and its imminent injunction to look on the bright side. Apart from tales of individual bravery, endeavour or luck, most newspaper stories are designed to enrage, upset, frighten and otherwise encourage all those negative emotions of jealousy and territoriality which we seem to relish, which is why papers published by the types who ask, 'Why can't there be more good news in the papers?' invariably fail.

But the truth is that in the developed world, for most of us, most of the time, life is as good as it ever could be and infinitely better than it was for any generation preceding ours. As a teenager, I was, like millions of others, taken with the Utopianism of William Morris's *News from Nowhere* and the description of a society where equality and social justice prevailed and as a result fear, anger, jealousy and the rest of it fell away. It wasn't just that everyone in that impossible world had plenty to eat, a roof over their head and fulfilling work, but that they never woke up feeling grumpy, never envied anyone else their greater happiness, never suffered, in short, from the iniquities not of economic distribution but those of serotonin levels and pain thresholds.

Yes, I know it's easy for me in the soft south to say it, and I know that there is real poverty and deprivation in the country, that the income gap is widening and the distribution of the country's wealth is getting less equitable by the day. And yes, I know too that it's no comfort to the freezing pensioner or the confined single mother at the end of her tether to know that three or four generations ago their lives would have been regarded by the freezing and confined masses as normal or even comparatively desirable. But the fact remains that for the first time in the history of our species, the vast majority of us in the West have more than enough to eat, somewhere relatively warm to live, the ability to move ourselves around the country and even the world as the fancy takes us, a sufficiency of resources with which we can entertain and distract ourselves.

I understand why when the Rowntree Trust reports on poverty in Britain it annoys *Daily Mail* readers (or, more usually, writers) by including a TV and video recorder in the list of essentials without which normal life isn't considered possible, but I can't bring myself to believe that the reason for most of the unhappiness in the country has to do with economic imbalance as much as it does with some innate need for a couple of portions of discontent as part of our psyche's emotional diet.

But even if you can't agree with that as a description of the country as a whole, let's look at it as a description of you and me, that part of society which reads lengthy essays in broadsheet Sunday newspapers and which, by that definition, has enough superfluous income to afford the paper and enough superfluous time to read it.

The other week, I wrote in this paper about alternative medicine. Briefly put, I was, and am, against it because I think it doesn't work on real organic illness. I don't want to rehearse that argument again here, but what I didn't point out in the piece is that the boom in alternative medicine has little to do with the failure of orthodox remedies to cure serious diseases – the vast majority of people with heart conditions or cancer or what have you still, quite rightly, submit to the orthodoxy – but with the alternativists' claims to be able to deal with illnesses which orthodox doctors can't diagnose, let alone treat.

They are, if you like, the luxury illnesses, the illnesses which can be afforded by a society with too little to worry about. In my pre-cancerous, hypochondriacal days, I was forever presenting my GP with vague symptoms of even vaguer illnesses, being sent off for blood tests, investigations to see whether my fluttering heartbeat was a sign of something more organically entrenched than a mere fondness for too many cigarettes, late nights and dodgy social situations. They are the illnesses which result from over-expectation, from the belief that we can feel happy, comfortable, positive, motivated all the time. But to feel that good that often you have to be pretty stupid in that way that stupidity so often manifests itself, as a lack of imagination.

But because most of us aren't stupid and do have enough imagination to posit a world beyond our immediate and personal space and time, we create worries which previous generations wouldn't have had time for. It's no coincidence, for instance, that animal rights as anything but the most intellectual of concepts has arrived as a popular movement only with postwar prosperity. Only the rich, with their Gore-Tex and Polar Fleeces can afford to be sniffy about animal skins; in polar societies where you skin a seal or die of hypothermia the options for animal liberationists are more limited.

Or we worry about televised violence but rarely stop to consider that ours is one of a handful of recent generations which only sees that sort of violence on television. I, for instance, have never seen a dead body in, as it were, the flesh, but I doubt if my four-times great-grandfather escaping the pogroms of Russia could have said that, or even somebody brought up in a big city during the war. My children have seen only the most cartoon-like violence and are nonetheless shocked by it: a London child two hundred years ago would have lived in a town surrounded by death, disease, prostitution, violence and poverty on a level we can only imagine.

It's the same with politics generally. Until relatively

recently, mass political movements were still about basic rights of food, shelter, education and self-sufficiency. The reason fewer people vote these days, or turn up to political meetings, is that for the vast majority of us those rights have been fulfilled. The nearest thing we had to a political rally this year had nothing to do with the rights of man or human suffering or any of the subjects which my forebears – or even my younger self – would have recognised as the sort of thing which brought a country to its knees; no, it was about the price of petrol, and although at one level it was about the conditions that lorry drivers and farmers operate under, for the most part it was about how much it costs us to drive in our own cars into work every day.

The nonsense of the campaign as a chapter in the movement for human rights became most apparent when the lorry drivers hijacked the spectre of the Jarrow March to push their essentially petit-bourgeois message. But then, that's the nature of modern politics and the only time you'll see the old political icons these days is in adverts for mobile phones or foreign holidays where phrases like 'Join the revolution!' and 'Cry freedom!' are bandied about for a generation which knows nothing of their provenance. Just as we have luxury illnesses to replace the real ones, so we now have luxury politics.

All of which seems to have distracted me from the chirpiness I promised and, more importantly, the answer to the editor's question.

And the answer is this:

This is what it's all about. It's about reading a paper on a Sunday morning while you're thinking about whether you can be arsed to go to the neighbours' New Year's Eve party tonight. It's about getting angry with me for having different opinions from yours or not expressing the ones you have as well as you would have expressed them. It's about the breakfast you've just had and the dinner you're going to have. It's about the random acts of kindness which still, magically, preponderate over acts of incivility or nastiness. It's about rereading *Great Expectations* and about who's going to win the 3.30 at Haydock Park. It's about being able to watch old episodes of *Frasier* on satellite TV whenever we want, having the choice of three dozen breakfast cereals and seven brands of virgin olive oil at Sainsbury's. It's about loving and being loved, about doing the right thing, about one day being missed when we're gone.

And that's all it's about. It isn't about heaven and hell or the love of Christ or Allah or Yahveh because even if those things do exist, they don't have to exist for us to get on with it.

It is, above all, I suppose, about passing time. And the only thing I know that you don't is that time passes at the same rate and in much the same way whether you're going to live to forty-eight or 148. Why am I happy? Because I'm alive. And the simple answer to the question 'What the hell is the point of it all?' is this is the point of it all. You aren't happy? Yes you are: this, here, now, is what happiness is. Enjoy it.

Observer

13 JANUARY 2001

ANGER

THIS WEEK OI 'as, as the yokel on *The Fast Show* has it, bin mainly shoutin' at people. Which, in my situation, means writing very quickly and in capitals in my notebook so that the pen pierces the paper and the object of my anger can't read what it is I'm angry about, which makes me angrier still and the whole thing dissolves into madness.

I went, for instance, to Curry's to buy a new vacuum cleaner because the old one choked itself to death on the Christmas detritus. After some consumer nonsense of the so-why-the-hell-do-you-keep-it-on-display-when-you-don't-have-it-in-stock? variety, I chose one of the less gaudily purple Dyson models because, although the things always look as if they've been made from a kit on somebody's kitchen table, they are A Product of British Ingenuity, and worthy of our indulgence. I got out my credit card. 'Postcode?' the salesman said. 'You don't need my postcode,' I wrote. 'It's for the guarantee,' he said. 'No, it's not,' I wrote.

'The receipt is proof of purchase; you don't need my address if it breaks, do you?'

Of course, if Curry's or Dyson really want my address they can find it easily enough. It's just that I'm on as many computer databases as I need to be and at that moment was irritated by the suggestion that I could only buy the damned cleaner if I volunteered my address so that somebody in marketing could more precisely work out the demographics of Hoover-buying. 'Sorry, sir: I must have the address.' I have the notepad by me now: the scribbled ghost of the phrase, 'Do

271

you want my business or not?' can be seen chiselled into the paper six pages deep. And would you believe it? The man turned down a £250 sale rather than leave the address box empty. So I went to Selfridges and bought a German Miele and not a word about addresses was spoken.

And then the next day I went to my bank to draw some money out from a hole in the wall. I'd just tapped in the number when a polite woman and two men in Edgware Road Middle Eastern garb stepped forward and pressed the cancel button. 'You mustn't use this machine,' one of the men said. 'She has just lost her card in there. It is a broken machine.' I turned back to the cash machine and sure enough it had swallowed my card and sat there grinning and asking for the next customer.

I slammed through the door of the bank and scribble-shouted, 'Your cash machine has just eaten my card!' at a cashier. She knew what had happened: people's cards get eaten when they try and take out more money than they have. It would, she said, eventually be returned by my branch. No, I screamed: there's something wrong with the machine: it ate the card of the woman in front of me, too. My account is full of money. I want my card back now. The cashier gave the standard speech about waiting until the machine was emptied at the day's end, and the card being sent back to my branch and all of that, and by the end of it I was piercing my note-book with threats of moving my account from Lloyds. I'd got as far as 'I'd like to see . . .' when she said, patiently, sweetly, 'Would you like to see the manager?', who turned up, toler-antly watched me shout some more and proceeded to look in the innards of the machine for my card.

Which wasn't there. Where it was, it turned out, was down the road at the local Abbey National, where the three solici-tous Middle Eastern characters were extracting £500 from my account. There are few things as embarrassing as a policeman supplying the punchline to the crime story you're telling him and 'I suppose they told you the machine wasn't working, did they?' ranks up there with 'I suppose you left the keys in the car while you went to pay for the petrol, then' as a euphemism for 'If the public weren't quite so congenitally stupid we'd be out of a job.'

I made my statement and then sought out the manager, who, in five minutes flat, had ascertained where the card had gone, brought me a cup of tea, got the police round and made sure I wasn't out of pocket as a result of the scam. I thanked him and apologised for shouting. He looked down at my notebook and smiled. 'Were you shouting?' he said. 'I didn't realise.'

The Times Magazine

27 JANUARY 2001

DONOR CARDS

IT WOULD BE falsely modest of me to pretend that I didn't realise that this column hasn't garnered me a certain sort of modest celebrity and that while I'm no Keith Chegwin or Craig out of *Big Brother*, there are certain circles where if you say 'John Diamond' the response will be, 'You mean the bloke who writes that column about his neck in *The Times*?' But until I got the call from the editor the other day I didn't realise how insanely far it had gone.

The Central Office of Information, I'm told, phoned up this paper's advertising department to buy space in the magazine in which to place an official government advertisement. I say 'I'm told' because, like all journalists, I like to preserve the fiction that newspapers are maintained entirely by the money you pay to read what we have to say about the world and its ways, and that the pages subsidised by Dixons and PC World and all those companies flogging sofas are mere ornaments published to give the readerly eye a rest in between scoops. The COI, you will know, is that department charged with bringing the valiant work of the government to the notice of the masses, and the department which, *inter alia*, tells *Times* readers that Coughs and Sneezes Spread Diseases or that Walls Have Ears or whatever the latest campaign is.

What it wants to tell you this time is that the gentlemanly thing to do when you fall under a bus is to be retrieved from the gutter with an organ donor card in your wallet giving permission for your corneas and kidneys to be passed on, as if in some physiological relay race, to somebody who is currently stumbling around blind and kidneyless.

What better message could there be for a government to pass on to those who elected it. True, I don't carry a donor card myself because it got nicked along with the rest of the contents of my wallet some four years ago and I've yet to get round to replacing it. It's possible, of course, that the thief who used my credit cards for the few hours before I realised they were gone has himself fallen under a bus and his kidneys are sitting beneath a grateful third party's ribs masquerading as my own. In any case I'll let this column serve as *carte blanche* for my organs to be used, *post mortem*, for any purpose the surgeons see fit – feeding the hospital cat included.

But, as is so often the case these days, I digress. The COI wants to place an ad in this magazine promoting donor cards, and more specifically it asked if the ad could be placed opposite this column. Not acknowledging the existence of the ad department, I only have this information second-hand, but the way I heard it their theory was that the sort of people who read this column – i.e., you – are the sort most likely to be susceptible to entreaties to carry organ donor cards. It is what I understand they call in the trade 'product placement' – the equivalent of Coca-Cola paying good money for Arnie or Sly to be seen drinking their product in their newest Hollywood offering on the basis that if you see a muscle-bound multi millionaire with a dodgy accent drinking Coke, you will want to drink it too.

The editor e-mailed me to ask if I minded sitting next to an organ donor ad, and of course I don't. As causes go it's a good one, and in any case I was flattered. So would you be. Just imagine: a brainstorming session in Whitehall, a dozen civil servants charged with increasing heart–lung transplants by 2.4 per cent before third fiscal quarter '01, and whose name do they pick to do the job? Exactly! 'We're after dead people,' they cry. 'Let's get Diamond on the case! His is the name which has become synonymous with cheery death.' And what more surreal, what more bizarre sort of celebrity can you imagine than that? Not that I'd encourage anyone in need to go for my particular heart–lung combination, of course.

The ad will appear next week or possibly the week after that, and because that week I'll probably be talking about something completely different, and because if I didn't mention it some of you were bound to write in and ask if anyone here had noted the proximity of it to me, I thought I ought to tell you in advance. Donor cards? I'm all for them. Put me down for a tongue and a couple of lungs, will you?

The Times Magazine

28 JANUARY 2001

DOCTORS ARE MUCH SAFER THAN

THEY SEEM

THESE THINGS HAPPEN, you know? An eighteen-year-old leukaemia patient turns up on your ward for his chemotherapy and can you remember for the life of you where the damn stuff goes? Is this the one which goes in the vein or the other one which goes in the – er, lots of little bones, run down the back, stumpy bit on the end with the funny name? Spine! That's the one! Spine, vein, vein, spine. Whatever. Bung the needle in: the contents will get wherever it's meant to get in the body one way or another, right? Except – what d'ye know? Turns out to be one of those pesky cytotoxins that if you stick it in the guy's back – pffft! Writhing agony for a bit and then all over. Dead as a dead thing. Never mind. Send the next patient in, will you, Miss Prendergast?

The poor leukaemic teenager made his appearance in the papers on Wednesday. On Tuesday it had been the turn of the anaesthetist who returned to work after having his banishment by the General Medical Council rescinded by the Privy Council, and went on to commit sundry acts of operating theatrical mayhem – including losing to gangrene a few fingers, lately the property of a woman in for a back operation – before being struck off again a couple of years later. And on Thursday we were introduced to the GP who managed not to spot the football-sized tumour in the pelvis of a young girl (now deceased), but who was allowed by the GMC to keep his licence to practise.

Add to that the most recent revelations concerning Harold Shipman's attempts to cleanse Cheshire, or whatever it was that he thought he was doing when the voices spoke to him, and you have, more or less, fixed the current standing of doctors in the public imagination. If they don't actually set out to kill you on purpose then they'll do it by accident.

It's a view which fits in with our new, consumerist view of healthcare. We don't like doctors because they tell us what to do rather than giving us the choice that consumerism demands we have. If medicine were a truly modern and democratic practice then we wouldn't get a prescription from a GP but a menu of options, with something for every medical taste and pocket, and never mind that few of us have even the most basic knowledge we need to choose between what's on offer.

We used to like doctors, of course, or have some respect for them at least, but that was in the days when there was some communal respect for people who knew things we didn't. Now all such esoteric knowledge is regarded as suspect, as somehow unjust. If knowledge is power and power should, in a democracy, be in the hands of us all, then it follows that knowledge should be in our hands too. Except that – wouldn't you know it? – knowledge and skill are so terribly hard to acquire. It takes years stuck away in libraries, mugging things up from textbooks in poky lodging rooms, living on a pittance, being bored when you could be down at the pub.

And because it's taken for granted now that anything which is inequitable must be bad, we simply downgrade the esteem in which those who have special skills, special knowledge, are held. We like nurses, for instance, because they don't get paid much, tend to use the same pubs as we do and we know that if we were willing to spend a couple of weeks learning how to give an enema or wipe the spittle off a geriatric's jowls we could do the job as well. But doctors? No: all those long Latin words and that funny writing. How can they not be suspect?

And the suspicion feeds itself and is, in turn, fed by the press. It turns out, for instance, that, according to the Department of Health, ten patients have been killed by having their chemotherapy syringed into their spine by mistake since 1985, which is ten too many of course and probably all of those deaths were highly preventable, but it still works out at five-eighths of a death a year, which, with an incidence of over a quarter of a million cancer diagnoses in the country each year, isn't what you'd call a widespread outbreak. Incompetent anaesthetists? I'm sure there are plenty of them working away in our hospitals – but sufficiently few so that when one does get caught it makes headlines in the national press.

On the radio the other day there was an earnest discussion based on the premise that the Harold Shipman case was symptomatic of something which worried British health consumers. Everyone round the table accepted this gobbet of hyperbole as a reasonable presumption, as if Shipman were representative of some greater mass-murdering proclivity among doctors. It's nonsense of course: the last murdering doctor most people can bring to mind is Crippen, getting on for a hundred years ago. But it fitted in with the feeling that doctors have exclusive knowledge about our inner workings; how can they not want to use that knowledge – that power – to their own ends?

And whistling to summon up my hobby horse here, the only ones benefiting from this scaremongering are the alternative quacks: the medical democrats whose knowledge is so basic you can find it all in a Teach Yourself book at the local Waterstone's.

Sunday Telegraph

10 FEBRUARY 2001

FROM YOUR WAR CORRESPONDENT

THERE ARE TIMES when I feel I'm covering a long and particularly futile war. I use the analogy purely journalistically rather than medically: I've always avoided the usual bellicose references to suffering an illness. I am not fighting cancer – although my doctors are, I hope – nor battling with cancer, nor involved in a campaign, a skirmish, or a punch-up with it. It's the reporting itself that's warlike. In wars the cycle of stories is always much the same: there was fighting, people got killed, the fighting stopped, the fighting started again, some more people got killed, and then it stopped . . . That's how war is.

Cancer, too, it turns out. The first time I mentioned my cancer, it was, as far as I was concerned at least, big news. There was so much to say, so much to marvel at, so much to appal. But over the past coming-up-to four years, the novelty has worn off and the story has become: cancer comes, surgery, cancer goes, nothing happens, cancer comes back, radiotherapy . . . and so on through, so far, diagnosis, seven operations, three lots of radiotherapy, some chemotherapy and various smaller medical interventions. And so when I say, 'Guess what? The cancer is back,' that's almost all I have to say. It's been back before. If it goes, then it will come back again. It's what cancer does. What my cancer does, at least.

It's become so mundane that I thought of not mentioning it this week, save as a footnote to a tale of ordinary life. (Not that life is particularly ordinary at the moment. Five days a week, twelve hours a day, we are currently sharing our house

– all of our house – with the dozen production-crew members working on Nigella's next television series, four of whom seem to be tasked with setting lights and obscuring windows and generally making the kitchen look unlike our kitchen, or any other kitchen, and thus making it look more like our kitchen for the screen. All else aside, it means I walk around shielding my face from the roaming camera like some sex offender trying to slip through the photographers in front of the court house. I don't know why. In certain circumstances I'm still happy to go in front of the cameras. It's just that, with the breathing tube and the sundry scars, I have to psych myself up for it more than I'm able to when I'm a background character in my own house.) I digress, for to be strictly accurate I might be overstating the case regarding the returned cancer. Short-winded as I've been for the past couple of months, I suddenly became windless almost to the point of becalmment. We went to the hospital, I had an X-ray, I gave it to Martin Gore, my oncologist, who rushed up to show it to somebody else, and then came back and told me about the abnormality. It's a wonderful medico-weasel word, is 'abnormality'. We can all cope with a bit of abnormality in our lives and, much of the time, I insist on it; it's lumps and pains and collapsing organs I have the problem with. Which is what the abnormalities usually turn out to be. After all, there is no such phrase as 'only an abnormality' in the medical dictionary.

So there is a slight chance that the abnormality in my lung may be an infection. Another infection. I'm on the sort of multiple antibiotics that I imagine they give to tubercular cows and I feel permanently queasy. The idea is that I stay on the drugs for a couple of weeks in the hope that when I go for my next scan, it turns out that the abnormality has been righted. But I can't pretend I believe that will happen. I'm an old hand at this: I know the symptoms. I know the difference between this sort of breathlessness and that sort, between the sort of bloody residues I get from a chafing tracheostomy tube, and those which I get from a tumour getting into its murderous stride.

As we got up to leave Martin Gore's office, I said, 'So what's your hunch, then?' expecting him to say, as doctors usually do, 'I don't know, let's see what the scan says in a fort-night.' But he said, with infinitely preferable honesty, 'My hunch is that it's tumour.' Mine, too.

The Times Magazine

24 FEBRUARY 2001

THE FINAL INSULT

STRANGELY, I DON'T much mind about losing the hair on my head for a while, but I'm annoyed that I'll be bald-chested.

My one great pride in all of this is that there are now medical schools where they use the book I wrote about being cancerous as a textbook to give apprentice doctors some idea of what it's like to be a patient. What greater compliment could anyone pay me? But then isn't it good news that these days doctors are trained in something more customer-orientated than just which rib goes where and how to nudge an errant kidney back into place? Still, though, I think there is one important lesson that all doctors could learn, or at least those doctors who expect one day to deal with the major-league illnesses, and I know the man to teach it to them.

What doctors need to know is how to bridge that two-second gap between opening the door of the room in which your terrified patient is waiting with his wife and speaking the first words. What do you do? Downcast eyes? Affected jollity? Thin, sympathetic smile? Pretend to be flicking through your notes as if they might have changed since you last looked down at them? Maintain a chatty conversation with the accompanying nurse then turn to the patient – rather as those afternoon television hosts pretend to be engrossed in conversation until they notice the camera is on them?

Believe me, I've had them all. And the best is my oncologist. I mean it. He'd just given me the news the other day and I found that the only thing I could write down in response was 'God, but you did that so well.' Which sounds sarcastic, but it absolutely isn't intended as such. After all, as I told you the other week, I was pretty certain what the news would be. We sat in the room, and the door swung open and he looked straight at me with no artfully composed face, and said, 'We're going to have to start treatment again,' as he walked in and sat down.

No messing. And especially no, 'How are you, then?' Why do doctors ask that? They've got the damned case-notes in front of them and they know how you are with rather more accuracy than you do. Sometimes they vary this: 'How are you feeling then?', to which the only answer is, 'Tell me whether the cancer's back and I'll tell you how I'm feeling.'

The cancer is back, of course. Small volume, slow-growing. Slow-ish, at least. It's here in the lung, and there in the lung too, and back in the neck as well. But I responded well – hah! – to chemotherapy last time, so next week I start chemotherapy again. Three lots of it at three-weekly intervals as a puking outpatient, and this time my hair will fall out, just like a real cancer patient's, and I'll have to start wearing one of those jokey baseball caps that child leukemia patients always wear when they have their pictures taken by the local paper.

When all this started coming up four years ago, a medically literate friend sat with me as I checked through the details of my cancer on the Internet. In those days it was going to be a titchy, low-grade sort of cancer, which would be scared off by its first sight of the radiotherapy machine. 'The great thing is', he said, 'you'll get just as much sympathy as if it were real cancer!' Oh, but how we chuckle at such small ironies these days.

But baldness is one of the standard icons of real cancer, and the Marsden is always full of people in big hats and bad NHS wigs. When the oncologist told me about the hair loss, I thought of it only in terms of being bald (or, more honestly, balder), but as I write it occurs to me that the chemo won't distinguish between head hair and eyebrow hair or chest hair or in general reducing me to the state of an alopecic ten-year-old. Strangely, I don't much mind about losing the hair on my head for a while, but I'm annoyed that I'll be bald-chested. I know the modern vogue is for smooth men, and that a hairy chest is what you have if you wear a medallion and drive a Ford Capri, but I am of an era when chest hair spelt masculinity, and those associations stay in the mind long after rational consideration has kicked in. As emasculating as have been most of the treatments I've had, this will be the one, I think, which most adds insult to injury.

The Times Magazine